EAT
Yourself
SLIM

The World's BEST Method
to Lose Weight and Stay Slim

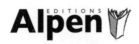

Exclusive copyrights:

Exclusive copyrights:
©Alpen Éditions
9, avenue Albert II
98000 Monaco
Tel: +377 97 77 62 10
Fax: +377 97 77 62 11
web: www.alpen.mc

Printed in Italy
ISBN: 978-2-35934-038-9

EAT
Yourself
SLIM

The World's BEST Method
to Lose Weight and Stay Slim

EDITIONS
Alpen

TABLE OF CONTENTS

PREFACE

Haven't you ever wondered why there are more and more obese people today than ever before even though calorie counting diets and exercise programs have been the norm for decades? Michel Montignac has asked the same question. And he has come to a very different conclusion than the scientists who study this paradoxical phenomenon.

Years ago, medical researchers discovered the link between obesity and changes to the secretion of the hormone insulin, which is associated with diabetes, arterial hypertension, and heart disease. Indeed, adult-onset diabetes (Type II) often goes hand-in-hand with excess weight. But is it the weight that causes diabetes, like so many doctors believe, or the other way around?

Michel Montignac has held the opposite view. Since the mid-1980s, he has argued that excess secretion of insulin, known as hyperinsulinism, was the cause, not the result, of obesity. Noting its debilitating effects on health, Montignac stressed that this hyperinsulinism was a direct result of the modern Western diet, which mainly consists of carbohydrates that increase insulin production, namely refined grains, potatoes, corn, and sugar. Montignac suggested that by eating carbohydrates low on the Glycemic index (GI) (those that don't excessively increase insulin levels), such as whole wheat and brown rice, the obese could not only lose weight, but also reduce their risk of diabetes and heart disease.

Initially, his message fell on deaf ears. Indeed, critics charged that the Montignac Method had never undergone scientific scrutiny. But in 1998, cardiologist Jean Dumesnil changed all that.

He and his colleagues at the Heart Institute at Laval Hospital in Quebec, Canada, studied the Montignac Method and concluded that it was more effective in helping people lose weight than other traditional diets. Dumesnil also showed that the Montignac Method had a favourable effect on cholesterol and insulin levels, which is beneficial to heart health.

Montignac has been further vindicated by Dr. Walter Willett's 1997 study at the Harvard School of Public Health in Boston. It showed that women who ate a low-glycemic, high-fibre diet had 2.5 times less risk of developing diabetes.

Michel Montignac, long ridiculed for his hypothesis and method, is now seeing his theories affirmed by legitimate scientific studies. I am obviously thrilled to see his ideas triumph, as I have personally always believed in them. But let us hope that, in the media storm that is bound to erupt over his challenge to classic theories of nutrition, Michel Montignac will prevail and be seen as one of the pioneers of a major transformation in the way we eat—all this in time for the third millennium. Michel Montignac was the first nutritionist in the word to introduce the glycemic index concept in the weight loss area.

Since the launching of his first book in 1986, his nutritional recommendations have widely inspired most best selling diet books.

Professor Hervé Robert
Doctor of Nutritional Sciences
University of Paris

PREAMBLE

Obesity is one of the major health problems confronting world population today. For decades, obesity has been considered an exclusively American problem. But now we are told by the World Health Organization that it has developed into a world-wide epidemic – a major health risk that is the underlying cause of many acute illnesses, such as diabetes and cardiovascular disease. Since the middle of the twentieth century, nutritionists and dieteticians have told us we are fat because we eat too many calories and because we do not exercise enough. This is why they have recommended us to follow a low-calorie diet, by eating less and reducing our intake of high calorie fatty food.

For half a century, nutritionists have encouraged us to eat low fat diets that are, by definition, nutritionally unbalanced. However, much to the surprise of the medical world, since the beginning of the nineteen-nineties, many scientific surveys and epidemiological studies have shown that though people in the West have decreased their calorie intake mainly by eating less fat, since 1960 the prevalence of obesity has increased fourfold.

Moreover, several medical studies have shown that fatty calories are far less involved in weight gain than what was originally thought. This has led some to suggest that carbohydrates are the real cause of weight gain, because they cause a sharp rise in blood sugar levels. This is due to the extra secretion of insulin into the bloodstream that they promote, causing any fat or sugar in the form of glucose to be stored in our body cells rather than burned as energy, and resulting in weight gain and a feeling of fatigue.

This is why some nutritionists like Dr. Atkins recommend a low-carb diet. However, although low carb diets are good at helping us lose weight, they have some major drawbacks. They are nutritionally unbalanced and force the body to get its energy requirements from muscle and fatty mass, thereby losing weight. This sort of diet however, imposes considerable strain on our metabolism, is dangerous, and cannot be sustained long-term without risk to our health.

The lack of carbs in our diet also leads us to compensate by eating more fat usually saturated animal fat. This is also dangerous, because too much saturated fat significantly increases the risk of cardiovascular disease, by raising LDL cholesterol, triglycerides, and hypertension to dangerous levels.

The Montignac Method, devised by French nutritionist Michel Montignac, achieves the same degree of weight loss achieved by low-carb diets, but manages to do so by maintaining a nutritionally balanced diet that is not only healthy, but is also very effective in helping combat cardiovascular disease.

How can this be? Well, put quite simply, it comes in the wake of Montignac's discovery in the early 1980's, that hyperinsulinism – not calories– is the real cause of weight gain. For almost 25 years now, Michel Montignac has devoted himself to the task of demonstrating to the world that hyperinsulinism is the underlying cause of obesity – not the other way around, as is still believed by many in the medical profession today. Not all carbohydrates have the same metabolic effects. Some may indirectly induce a high insulin response that will transform energy into fat reserves, but others do not and will not therefore cause us to put on weight.

The carbs that do not cause us to put on weight, Michel has called "good" carbohydrates: those that do, he has called "bad" carbohydrates – a distinction later extended to include "good" and "bad" fats, because of their ability to help combat or promote cardiovascular disease. Later still, Michel discovered that some fats could even help us lose weight.

The Montignac Method has become widely known as "the good carb and fat diet" – the only diet that leads to dramatic weight loss, is totally balanced, and does not require us to crash diet or starve ourselves. Its basic message is simple: to achieve our correct body weight, we must learn to distinguish between "good" and "bad" food within the three main categories of carbohydrates, fats, and proteins.

Already well known in America, the Montignac Method is famous both in Western and Eastern Europe, as well as in other areas such as the Middle East and Australia. More than 20 million Montignac books have been sold worldwide and sales continue to grow at an exponential rate, whilst the list of well-known super-chefs and celebrities committed long-term to the method, increases by the day. I am therefore proud and happy to present to you, the last version of this world wide famous diet.

The publisher

FOREWORD

Excessive weight, unfortunately, is part of today's society. It is a direct result of civilization. Primitive societies rarely exhibit obesity. The animal kingdom is also unaffected by obesity as long as species live in their natural environments. Only domesticated animals suffer from it.

Overweight people usually live in the most evolved societies. Indeed, the higher the standard of living, the more obesity there is. The story has remained the same throughout history. Not too long ago, being overweight was highly regarded. It not only symbolized social success, but it also connoted good health.

Today, we no longer think of obesity as being healthy. In fact, we revere thinness not only as a new measure of beauty, but also because we are now more aware how extra pounds can undermine our physical well-being. Obesity can be downright dangerous. Nowhere is obesity more evident than in North America, where it is reaching epidemic proportions, although it is climbing to comparable levels in a number of other countries, notably Russia. All indications point to poor eating habits and the notoriously bad North American diet. In fact, obesity is also appearing at a frightening rate in countries where North American food has been exported.

Contrary to what certain doctors often suggest, obesity is not a result of fate. While obesity may run in families, poor eating habits are also to blame. Without recognizing this important point, we would be concentrating on the effect (the weight) instead of the cause. That's why traditional diets fail. Instead of looking to fad diets to lose pounds, we would be better off to analyze why we gain weight. Instead of blindly following lists of ready-made menus, counting calories or measuring food, we should look at how our body functions and in what ways it assimilates different types of food.

The process of losing weight and keeping it off begins with education. Before beginning to put the principles described in this book into action, you'll learn three important points that form the foundation of the Montignac Method. First, you'll become aware of the deplorable eating habits we have acquired over several decades. Our consumption of refined foods such as sugar and white bread wreaks havoc on our metabolism. This is what causes obesity and poor health. Next, you'll find out how our metabolism and digestive system operate. Finally, you'll learn about the nature of food, its individual properties, and the food groups to which it belongs.

Over the last few years, every time I was asked how I have maintained my slim build, I have always answered, "By eating in restaurants and going to business dinners." People smiled, but I knew that they weren't really convinced. That's because most people blame their excess weight on the fact that they can't control their food intake at family, social, or professional functions.

Most likely, you have already tried a number of current popular diets. You may have also noticed that the methods often contradict each other and produce temporary, if any, results. What's more, you may have found it practically impossible to fit these diets into daily life. Even at home, they are so restricting that you quickly lose interest and become discouraged. The result: you're still overweight. I've been there, too. At the age of eight, I was already overweight. Obesity is hereditary on my father's side. He was overweight as were many of the men in his family. In my pre-adolescence, I was often mocked by my friends, who were naturally thinner than I was. In the years that followed, I enjoyed a reprieve. I was lucky enough to grow tall very quickly, which translated into a break in my weight-gain. But as soon as I turned 25, the extra pounds progressively reappeared, despite constant exercise and the food restrictions I placed on myself at the time. Ten years later in 1980, I found myself 35 pounds (16kg) overweight.

That's when I took a position in the European bureau of a large American pharmaceutical company. From then on, I travelled all the time and my visits to the U.S. branch offices often consisted of meetings centred around food. What's more, when I was in Paris, I had to wine and dine visitors at famous French restaurants as part of my public relations duties. Mind you, I didn't complain. But three months later, I found myself 11 pounds (5kg) heavier. The alarm bells went off inside my head. My weight was reaching a critical stage. Like all of us with weight problems, I tried to stop eating (especially fats) and exercise, just as all the diet books say you should do, but to no avail.

Just then I was fortunate enough to meet some nutrition researchers while on a trip to the United States who did not believe that the traditional methods of dieting worked. But they didn't offer me any alternatives. Struck by my obsession to lose weight, they gave me access to their science library full of studies on the subject of dieting. While reading the current research on diabetes, I found what I was looking for. The studies showed that 85 percent of diabetics were also obese. I saw immediately that the two conditions were linked. In one experimental study, Type II diabetics consumed only carbohydrates with a low glycemic potential. By doing so, these diabetics had substantially improved, and in some cases even suppressed their diabetes.

I figured that all I had to do, then, was try this nutritional approach to see if it could have a positive effect on weight loss. The result was amazing. In very little time, I had lost a favourable amount of weight. So I decided to delve more deeply into the matter, which was relatively easy for me to do since I worked in the field of science.

In a brief few months, I dropped a total of 35 pounds (16kg) by eating normally without restricting my food intake. Instead, I simply chose to eat certain foods and not others. This made it easier to eat out at restaurants, at dinner parties or office functions. By reading this book, you will come to understand how I was able to permanently eliminate a very serious weight problem by choosing the right foods in unlimited quantities and without having to do any additional exercise.

Everyone noticed the difference in just a matter of months and they wanted to know how I had achieved my success. My colleagues urged me to write down my formula—which took all of ten pages. But it did not end there. They continually bombarded me with questions. Everyone wanted to know how I was able to lose weight and still eat. I tried, as much as possible, to patiently explain the basic principles, but that was not always sufficient. Mistakes were made, and that, unfortunately compromised their results.

This book therefore is a guide, which will help you to understand my Method and how I arrived at it. The book will attempt to:

• demystify current notions of dieting by persuasive arguments that will convince you to abandon them as legitimate.

• provide fundamental scientific explanations for metabolism and how it affects weight gain.

• lay out simple guidelines along with their scientific validity.

For the past few years, with the advice of professionals, I have observed, researched, tested, and experimented with my Method. Today I feel confident that I have discovered and elaborated on an effective and easy method to put into practice. You will learn that we don't gain weight because we eat too much, but because we eat poorly. You will learn to manage your food intake just as one manages a budget. Finally, you will learn to eat better without starving.

But I do not call my Method a diet. Rather, it is a new way of eating, maintaining your weight while enjoying your food at home, at a social function or in a restaurant. You will be pleasantly surprised to learn that by adopting these new nutritional principles, you will find, as if by magic, a physical and intellectual vitality that you thought you had lost long ago.

Here's the reason why: your lack of energy can be traced to certain bad food habits. By adopting a few fundamental nutritional principles that are easy to put into practice, you will be able to end your mid-day slumps and discover optimal vitality. Even if you are not overweight, the Method and its principles are still important for developing good diet habits. In any case, you will discover a new energy to live your personal and professional life to the fullest. And you may even notice that if you have chronic digestive problems, they, too, will disappear.

While I love good French cuisine in general, wine, and chocolate in particular, I did not intend to copy the style of other excellent gourmet guides. Just the same, I confess to being tempted to do so because I find it difficult to dissociate nourishment from pleasure and simple cooking from gastronomical cuisine. Over the years, I have had the good fortune to dine at the best restaurants in the world and to shake hands with some of the most greatly admired and respected chefs.

Note:

The first version of this book came out in France in 1987. At that time, I couldn't find anyone to publish it because I was an unknown and I was challenging the way in which people were being told to lose weight. That's when I decided to publish my own book. In the beginning, it was only available by mail order. But since each book sold led to the sale of a dozen more, word of mouth boosted that amount to one million copies sold four years later. Today, more than six million copies have been sold in France, twenty million worldwide. It has been published in 45 countries and translated into 26 languages.

Since the publication of this book, its nutritional message has been enriched and refined, not only by the suggestions of my readers, but also from the observations made by a great number of doctors who now prescribe the Method. During all these years, I have personally dedicated most of my time and revenue to pursuing these research efforts so as to present an even clearer message. In some ways, my harshest critics have forced me to scientifically prove that my Method works, despite the obvious weight-loss success by thousands of people. Today, we can point to the work and observations of researchers in their publications (Bibliography) on the Montignac Method, whose positive results fulfilled our greatest dream.

CHAPTER 1:
THE CALORIE MYTH

The idea of basing weight loss on a low-calorie diet is, in my opinion, the most misleading proposition of 20th century science. It is the most simplistic and dangerous "hypothesis", without real scientific foundation. Yet it has governed the way we eat for more than half a century. Take a look around you. Most of the people who relentlessly count calories are invariably those who are overweight. With a few rare exceptions, every popular diet introduced over the last few decades has essentially been based on reducing calories. This has been unfortunate. Long-term weight loss is not possible using that method, not to mention the dangerous side effects that can occur. It seems impossible to change this trend because it has been so ingrained in the way we look at food and weight loss.

THE ORIGIN OF THE CALORIE THEORY

In 1930, two American doctors from the University of Michigan put forward their hypothesis that obesity was the result of a diet too "rich" in calories, rather than due to a deficiency in metabolism. They conducted a study on human requirements for energy. If you consume more calories than you need, they said, the rest is stored as fat. Their study was based on a very limited number of observations. But even more importantly, the time period over which it was conducted was much too brief to provide a legitimate scientific basis.

Despite this, the published results were accepted as irrefutable, scientific truth. Yet some years later, the two researchers, troubled by the fuss made over their discovery, quietly expressed some serious reservations about the conclusions that had made them so successful. But their concerns went completely unnoticed. Their theory was already inscribed into the medical school curriculums of most western countries, and still today, it holds sway.

THE CALORIE THEORY: AN ILLUSION

A calorie is the amount of energy necessary to raise the temperature of one gram of water from 14° to 15°C. First of all, the human body needs energy to maintain a temperature of 38°C (98.6°F); this is its basic need. But the moment the body moves, even if it is only to sit up, pick up a fork, or express sounds, more energy is required. In order to eat, digest, and accomplish everyday movements, we again need more energy. But daily energy needs vary among individuals, ages, and genders.

Here is the calorie theory in a nutshell. If the energy needs of an individual are, for example, 2,500 calories a day, and he or she only takes in 2,000, a 500-calorie deficit will result. In order to compensate for this, the human body will draw on stored fats to make up for the deficit. This supposedly leads to weight loss. On the other hand, if an individual consumes 3,500 calories daily, even though he or she only needs 2,500, that person will have an excess of 1,000 calories that will automatically be stored in the form of fat. The theory, then, is derived from the assumption that, no matter what, energy can neither be created nor destroyed.

The formula comes from an equation that is directly inspired by Lavoisier's theory on thermodynamic law. At this point one might begin to wonder how prisoners of concentration camps were able to survive for nearly five years on 800 calories a day. If the calorie theory were true, then, the prisoners should have died after just a few months, having already used up their fat stores and muscle mass. In the same vein, why is it that some people who consume 4,000 to 5,000 calories a day don't gain weight?

If the calorie theory holds, these individuals should end up weighing 900 to 1,000 pounds (400 to 450kg) in just a few years. Last, but not least, why is it that those people who are constantly following a reduced-calorie diet are usually the ones who are overweight? Indeed, millions of these individuals literally gain weight while starving themselves.

THE CALORIE PARADOX

Granted, when someone starts on a calorie-reduced diet for the first time, they do lose weight. But it is temporary. And this is where the University of Michigan researchers went wrong. Their study was based on short-term observation only.

The process goes like this: Let's assume that an individual's recommended needs are at 2,500 calories and that, over an extended period of time, a supply of calories is designed according to those needs. If suddenly the ration of calories drops to 2,000, the body will, as a result, use up a quantity of stored fats equal to the deficit, and we will see weight loss.

On the other hand, if the subject then establishes his or her supply of calories at 2,000 instead of the original 2,500, the body, moved by its survival instinct, will very rapidly adjust its energy needs to the level of the supply. Now that it is only being provided with 2,000 calories, it will only consume 2,000. Weight loss, therefore, will be abruptly interrupted.

But the body's response doesn't stop there. Its survival instinct will push for greater caution, so much so that it will create reserves. If, from then on, it is provided with only 2,000 calories, well then, it will again cut back its energy needs to, for example, 1,700 and then store the 300-calorie difference as fat reserves. Thus we get the inverse result of the one we were looking for because, even though one might be eating less, he or she is going to progressively gain the weight back. In fact, the human being, unfailingly moved by his or her survival instinct, behaves no differently than a dog who, when fed on an irregular basis, begins to bury its food, building up reserves even though it's starving.

Furthermore, we must acknowledge that calculations of calories are always theoretical and even approximate for the following reasons: from one chart or table to the next, the calorie-count for a single food can vary substantially.

THE RAVAGES OF WEIGHT-LOSS

The chart below shows the before and after scenario of a person who follows four diets with progressively reduced calorie-intakes, from 3,000 to 800 calories a day.

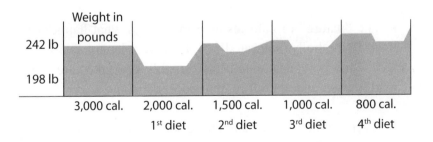

According to Dr. J.P Ruasse, this curve shows how successive low-calorie diets lead to a resistance to weight loss, and eventual obesity.

The caloric content of some foods fluctuates based on whether the foods are eaten raw or cooked, with or without added fats. Fat content (which causes the caloric content to vary) can fluctuate a great deal, from one piece of meat to the other. The fluctuation is dependent upon the way the animal was raised as well as the method in which it was cooked.

The calculation (theoretical) of calories never takes into consideration the rate of absorption of lipids and carbohydrates by the small intestine. This rate varies significantly based on the extent to which fibre is present in the meal. A significant proportion of fibre (notably soluble) can, in effect, substantially diminish the absorption of the said calories.

• Studies by L. Fakambi on fermented cheeses showed that if they are rich in calcium the calcium in the cheese retains a part of the fats that are not absorbed by the body. The corresponding calories then end up in the stool.

• The "nature" of calories also influences what happens to them in the body. Saturated fats, for example, are easily stored, while polyunsaturated fats (notably omega-3) are more readily used and, therefore, burned.

• Several studies (I. LeBlanc) have shown that levels of caloric expenditure due to food digestion (thermogenesis) differ greatly according to whether we eat the same number of calories in one single meal or in four to six spaced-out meals. The more the meals are broken up, the greater the caloric expenditure.

Finally, the simple calculation of calories does not take into consideration the time of day nutrients are absorbed. It has been shown that the absorption of carbohydrates, fats, and proteins varies according to different hours of the day and even according to the seasons (chronobiology). Their absorption also depends on the chemical environment that nutrients encounter when they reach the small intestine. The chemical environment depends on the kinds of nutrients, the order of their arrival and their volume. That's why any calculation of calories that doesn't take all of these additional factors into consideration borders on the absurd. How many of you have been victims of this unfounded theory of energy balance that has tried to convince us that the human body functions like a common furnace?

You have most likely come across overweight people in your group of friends who have tried starving themselves in order to lose weight. This is especially true among women. Psychiatrists' offices are filled with women for whom depression comes from following calorie-reduced diets. Upon entering the vicious cycle, these women rapidly become enslaved by it because they know that stopping will lead back to a weight gain even greater than the one with which they began.

Most members of the medical world know full well that their overweight patients fail to lose weight, but they secretly suspect their patients of not rigorously following their diets. Certain pseudo-professionals in the nutrition field have even organized group therapy sessions during which overweight people attest to their weight loss, which is praised with applause, while their weight gains are not discussed.

What's more, prescribing a 1,400-calorie diet without specifying which foods to eat, as do many traditional diets, is not sufficient. It all comes down to focusing on the notion that food is energy, without considering its nutritional value. Those in the medical field (save certain specialists) won't even question their basic understanding of nutritional value in this domain. In fact, nutrition is not an area that particularly interests doctors. I found that the ones who are interested in nutrition are those who had serious weight problems themselves.

The calorie theory has reached such a point that restaurant chains and neighbourhood diners post the number of calories for each item on their menus. Not a single week goes by that a number of women's magazines do not feature weight loss on their covers.

They offer the latest recipes by teams of professional dietitians who, basing them on the calorie theory, offer you meagre meals such as an orange for breakfast, half a piece of toast at 11:00, a chickpea at noon and an olive in the evening.

Unfortunately, it's often professional dieticians who are the worst offenders. In his book "La cuisine du bien maigrir" (published by Odile Jacob), Dr. Jacques Fricker, a well-known nutritionist in France, suggests low-calorie recipes calculated to the minutes detail. For example: crab meat— 199 calories (and not 200 or 201); sautéed veal milanaise— 299 calories (and not 300); poires soufflées—156 calories. Not one calorie more or less. It is absurd to pay so much attention to such an inexact science. Nevertheless, we need to look at the fact that calorie counting has been the accepted norm. There are two reasons:

1. The first is that a low-calorie diet often produces short term results. Food deprivation, on which the diet is founded, does lead to a certain amount of weight loss. But, as we have already seen, this result does not last. Not only will the dieter inevitably go back to his or her original weight, but also he or her will likely gain even more.

2. The second reason is that "low-calorie" has become big business. Professional dieticians, world-famous chefs, and major companies are all economic beneficiaries of the low-cal revolution.

The calorie theory is false, and now you know why. But that doesn't mean that you can be rid of it forever because, by now, it is so firmly embedded in your mind that you will continue to find yourself thinking along those lines for a long time. When we get to the eating Method that I recommend in this book, you may feel uncomfortable with the contradictions that you will face. If this is so, please feel free to review this chapter until it becomes clear to you.

CHAPTER 2:
THE DIFFERENT TYPES OF FOOD

If you want to take control of your diet, which is the key to maintaining a healthy weight, the first step is to learn to recognize the kinds of foods that you eat. This chapter may be a bit technical, but it is easily mastered. That's because you may already be familiar with the basics. But don't let that stop you from reading this chapter. It is essential to understanding how the Method works. Besides, what you think you may know may be erroneous. There are so many myths about foods that this chapter will debunk. So follow along, if only out of curiosity. Foods are edible substances that contain a variety of nutrients, such as proteins, fats, carbohydrates, vitamins, minerals, and trace elements. They also contain water and non-digestible materials, such as fibre.

PROTEINS

Proteins are the organic cells that form the foundation of living matter: muscles, organs, the brain, the skeletal structure, etc.

These proteins consist of simpler molecules called amino acids. Some amino acids are produced by the body, but mostly they are derived from food. Protein comes in two forms:

1. Animal: meats, fish, cheese, eggs, and dairy products

2. Vegetable: soy, almonds, hazelnuts, whole grains and certain legumes, such as beans and lentils

Ideally, you should consume proteins by drawing equally from vegetable as well as animal sources. But that is not always easy to do. Proteins are indispensable to the body. Their functions are:

• to build cells that produce energy after they are transformed into glucose (the Krebs cycle)

• to make certain hormones and neurotransmitters, a chemical substance released by nerve endings

• to build up nucleic acids, which are necessary for reproduction

A diet deficient in proteins can lead to serious side effects: muscle atrophy, immune deficiency, skin problems, etc. Children should eat about 60 grams of protein a day, while teens need about 90 grams. Adults, on the other hand, should eat a gram of protein for every kilogram of weight (2.2 lb.), totalling about 55 grams for women, and 70 for men. What's more, 15 percent of energy requirements should come from proteins.

However, you can consume more protein than recommended without serious consequences, up to 1.5 grams per day per kilogram, as long as you drink enough liquids to eliminate the waste generated by protein metabolism (uric acid, urea, lactic acid). In fact, greater protein intake can effectively help in your weight-loss phase. First, because its metabolism leads to greater energy expenditure than other foods. And second, because it causes you to feel fuller more quickly. According to Professor D. Tome, *"it seems that an adult's regulatory capacity allows him or her to adapt to a wide range of protein intake, between 0.6 and 2 grams per kg (2.2 lb.) per day, without major visible repercussions on overall health"* (Chole, doc. no. 45, Jan/Feb., 1998).

Except for eggs, animal or vegetable proteins alone do not provide the necessary balance of amino acids. The absence of one amino acid can limit absorption of other amino acids. Your diet must consist of proteins of both animal and vegetable origin. A diet based solely on vegetable proteins (vegetarianism) would be unbalanced. It would notably lack cysteine, causing brittle hair and nails. On the other hand, a vegetarian diet including eggs and dairy products can be completely balanced.

CARBOHYDRATES

Carbohydrates are molecules made up of carbon, oxygen, and hydrogen. They are metabolized into glucose, which is a major energy source for the body, especially because it is readily available. There are several types of carbohydrates with varying molecular structures:

Simple sugars

- glucose: honey and fruit

- fructose: honey and fruit

- galactose: milk

Double sugars

- saccharide (glucose + fructose): white sugar extracted from beets or sugar cane

- lactose (glucose + galactose): milk

- maltose (glucose + glucose): beer and corn

Complex sugars
starch, which contains hundreds of glucose molecules, found in:

- grains: wheat, corn, rice

- tubers: potatoes, yams, artichokes

- roots: rutabaga, carrots

- legumes: beans, lentils, chickpeas and soy beans

Slow" and "quick" sugar are:

For years, carbohydrates have been classified into "slow" and "quick" sugars. But this has been misleading, and even incorrect. The classification was based on how long we thought it took the body to absorb them: under the heading "quick sugars" were the simple and double sugars such as glucose and saccharide, found in refined sugar (from sugar cane or sugar beets), honey and fruit. Quick sugars were allegedly absorbed rapidly by the body soon after ingestion.

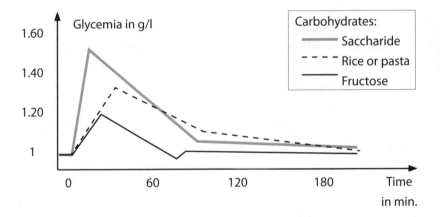

Conversely, "slow sugars" or complex carbohydrates, had to be chemically transformed into simple sugars (glucose) during digestion before they could be absorbed. This was notably true of starches, where glucose was released—or so we thought—slowly and progressively into the body. Today, this classification is completely outdated because it is based on erroneous thinking. Experiments have proven that, in effect, the complexity of the carbohydrate molecule does not determine the speed at which glucose is released and used by the body.

The glycemic peak, meaning the maximum absorption level, of all carbohydrates, eaten alone on an empty stomach, occurs in the same amount of time (around half an hour after the ingestion).

Instead of discussing assimilation speed, it would make more sense to study carbohydrates based on the rise in glycemia that they cause, that is, the quantity of glucose they cause the body to produce. Therefore, scientists (cf. Bibliography) have admitted that the classification of carbohydrates must be done based on their hyperglycemic potential, defined by the concept of the glycemic index (GI). But in order to help you understand the meaning of the glycemic index, which is one of the main tenets of the Montignac Method, we should first discuss the essential notion of glycemia.

WHAT IS GLYCEMIA?

Carbohydrates are an essential source of fuel for the body, especially the brain. That is the reason they are constantly present in the bloodstream. This presence is marked by what is called the glycemia level, which, on an empty stomach, normally works out to be about one gram of carbohydrates (sugar) per litre (approx. 1 quart) of blood.

If the level goes below this norm, the secretion of a pancreatic hormone, glucagon, re-establishes the normal level. When
we eat a carbohydrate, the absorption of corresponding glucose
will cause a rise in glycemia.

At first, glycemia will increase (more or less according to the
type of carbohydrate ingested) until it reaches a maximum,
which we call the glycemic peak.

The pancreas, an organ involved in the regulation of metabolic
processes, will then secrete another hormone, insulin, the objective being to eliminate the excess glucose in the blood and to
store it elsewhere in the body (the liver and muscles) in case it is
needed. Under the insulin's effect, the glycemia level becomes
lower until it finally returns to normal.

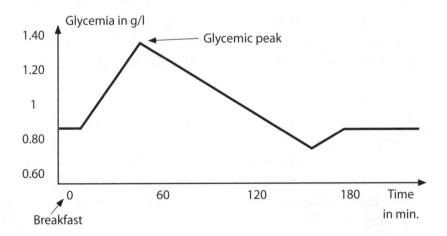

THE GLYCEMIC INDEX (GI)

The glycemic potential of each carbohydrate is defined by its glycemic ability and is measured by the GI, first established in 1976. It corresponds to the measure of the triangular surface of the hyperglycemic curve induced by carbohydrate ingestion. We arbitrarily give glucose an index of 100, which represents the triangular surface of the corresponding hyperglycemic curve. The GI of other carbohydrates, therefore, is calculated by the following formula:

$$\frac{\text{Triangular surface of tested carbohydrate}}{\text{Triangular surface of glucose}} \times 100$$

The GI rises according to the level of hyperglycemia. Thus, the higher the GI, the higher the hyperglycemia induced by the carbohydrate will be. It should be noted that industrial processing and methods of preparing and cooking carbohydrates can raise their GI (cornflakes 85, corn 70, instant potatoes 95, boiled potatoes 70).

We also know that it is not only the composition of starch (ratio of amylase to amylopectin), but also the amount of protein and fibre, and the quality of fibre in carbohydrate rich foods that cause their indexes to be either low or high (hamburger rolls 85, white bread or baguette 70 whole wheat bread 45, white rice 70 and brown rice 50).

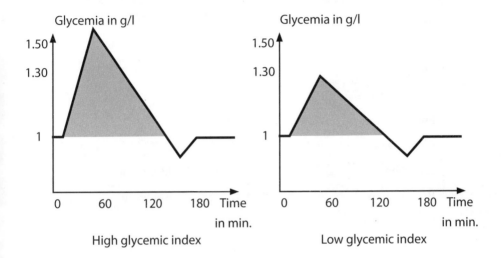

High glycemic index   Low glycemic index

In order to simplify matters, I propose dividing carbohydrates into two categories: "good carbohydrates" (having a low GI) and "bad carbohydrates" (having a high GI). In the following chapters this distinction will clarify for you the reasons why you are overweight.

BAD CARBOHYDRATES

These are the carbohydrates whose assimilation causes a significant rise in glucose in the bloodstream (hyperglycemia). These are: all forms of table sugar (either pure or in other foods, such as pastries) and all industrially refined carbohydrates, such as white flour, white rice and corn, as well as potatoes.

CARBOHYDRATES WITH HIGH GLYCEMIC INDEX

Maltose (beer)	110	Sugar (saccharose)	70
Glucose	100	Sweetened refined cereals	70
Modified starch	100	White bread (baguette)	70
Baked potatoes	95	White rice	70
Fried potatoes	95	Cooked beets	65
French fries	95	Corn	65
Rice flour	95	Jams (with added sugar)	65
Burger bread	85	Leavened brown bread	65
Cooked carrots	85	Raisins	65
Corn flakes, popcorn	85	Unpeeled boiled potatoes	65
Quick cooking rice	85	Bananas, melon	60
Puffed rice	85	Honey	60
Rice pudding	85	Long-grain rice	60
Cooked broad beans	80	Refined semolina	60
Mashed potatoes	80	Shortbread	55
Pumpkin	75	Well-cooked spaghetti	55
Watermelon	75	Sweet potato	50
Chips	70	Whole grain (brown) rice	50
Chocolate bars	70	Whole wheat pasta	50
Cookies	70	Long grain Basmati rice	50
Noodles, ravioli	70	Sweet potato	50
Peeled boiled potatoes	70	Whole grain (brown) rice	50
Sodas, cola soft drinks	70	Whole wheat pasta	50

CARBOHYDRATES WITH LOW GLYCEMIC INDEX

Whole cereals (no sugar added)	45	Dairy products	30
Whole grain rye bread	45	Brown, yellow lentils	30
Montignac pumpernickel	**40**	Pears	30
Montignac Basmati rice	**40**	Chickpeas	30
100% integral bread	40	Tomatoes	30
Dried figs, apricots	40	Soy vermicelli	30
Fresh fruit juices (no sugar added)	40	Dark chocolate (> 70% cocoa)	25
Ice-cream (with alginates)	40	Flageolet beans	25
Integral pasta *al dente*	40	Green lentils	25
Pumpernickel	40	Green vegetables	25
Red kidney beans	40	Split peas	25
Rolled oats	40	**Montignac sugar free jam**	**20**
Spaghetti *al dente*	40	Sugar-free marmalade	25
Montignac chocolate bars	**35**	**Montignac fructose**	**20**
Montignac biscuits	**35**	Eggplant	20
Dried white kidney beans	35	Fructose	20
Fresh apricot	35	Soya	20
Fresh garden peas	35	Onions	15
Green (string) beans	35	Peanuts, walnuts,	15
Maize/Indian corn	35	hazelnuts, almonds	15
Quinoa	35	Zucchini	15
Raw carrots	35	**Montignac low GI spaghetti**	**10***
Wild rice	35	* Scientifically calculated by an independent and registered laboratory	
Montignac Integral bread	**34***		

GOOD CARBOHYDRATES

Unlike bad carbohydrates, these are reducibly absorbed by the body, resulting in less of a rise in blood sugar (glycemia). These are: whole flours, brown rice, and particularly certain legumes such as lentils and kidney beans, most fruits and all vegetables that contain fibre (cabbage, broccoli, cauliflower, lettuce, green beans, leeks, etc.).

LIPIDS (OR FATS)

Lipids are complex molecules, more commonly known as fatty acids. There are two main lipid categories based upon their source:

1. **Animal lipids**: Meat, fish, butter, eggs, cheese, sour cream, etc.
2. **Vegetable lipids**: Peanut oil, olive oil, nut oils, margarine, etc.

Lipids are also classified into three categories according to the nature of their fatty acids:

1. **Saturated fats:** Meat, eggs and whole-fat dairy products (milk, butter, cream, cheese)

2. **Monounsaturated fats**: Olive oil, fats from goose and duck liver paté (foie gras)

3. **Polyunsaturated vegetable fats**: oil from seeds (mainly sunflower), oleaginous fruits

4. **Trans fat: margarine** (made by hydrogenating a polyunsaturated fat)

Polyunsaturated animal fats: lipids are essential to any diet. They provide storable energy that is readily available according to the body's needs. They control the formation of membranes, cells, and tissues, especially those of the nervous system. Fatty foods contain a number of vitamins (A, D, E, and K) and essential fats (linoleic acid and linolenic acid). They also aid in the manufacture of various hormones. It is best to eat all fats in moderation. Unfortunately, in our industrialized society, people tend to eat one kind of fat more often than others. These fats are found in fried foods, donuts and heavy sauces, which can cause a rise in cholesterol levels in the bloodstream.

There are two types of cholesterol: **HDL**, or "good" cholesterol, and **LDL**, or "bad" cholesterol. The objective is to maintain a normal total cholesterol level, keeping the level of good cholesterol (HDL cholesterol) as high as possible and the level of bad cholesterol (LDL cholesterol) as low as possible.

Not all lipids cause an increase in "bad" cholesterol, however. In fact, some even tend to significantly lower it.

To clarify the point, fats are classified into three categories:

Fats that raise cholesterol:

These are saturated fats found in meat, cold cuts, butter, cheese, lard, whole dairy products and palm oil, as well as trans fat.

Fats that are neutral with regard to cholesterol:

These are found in shellfish and eggs.

Fats that lower cholesterol:

These are found in vegetable oils (olive, rapeseed, sunflower, corn, etc.).

While fats derived from fish oil do not directly affect the metabolism of cholesterol, they do tend to prevent cardiovascular diseases by reducing triglycerides and hindering blood clots. Therefore, it is a good idea to incorporate fatty fish such as salmon, tuna, mackerel, herring, and sardines into your diet.

The method of weight loss I offer you in this book is essentially based on choosing between "good" and "bad" carbohydrates. If you have high cholesterol, you will be encouraged to choose between "good" and "bad" fats in order to prevent the risk of cardiovascular diseases[1] for good.

DIETARY FIBRE

Dietary fibre can be found in large quantities in carbohydrates with a low GI: vegetables, legumes, fruit, and unrefined grains. They are also found in unprocessed foods. Even though fibre provides no fuel, it is essential to good digestion.
It slows down the absorption of carbohydrates, resulting in a low glycemic response. There are two kinds of fibre:

1. Insoluble fibre (cellulose, hemicelulosa) helps the digestive tract push food efficiently through. When a diet is low in fibre, constipation usually results.

2. Soluble fibre (gum, pectin) limits digestive absorption, especially of lipids, and lowers the risk of atherosclerosis.

Fibre-rich foods are also rich in vitamins, trace elements[2], and mineral salts. Insufficient amounts of these can cause serious deficiencies. Fibre can also limit the toxic effects of certain chemical substances, such as additives and food colouring.

Some studies by gastroenterologists have shown that certain kinds of fibre can protect the colon and rectum from a number of diseases, especially cancers of the digestive system.

---

[1] Chapter 8 is devoted to hypercholesterolemia and its risk to cardiovascular health.
[2] Trace elements: metals or metalloids present in infinitesimal amounts in the human body, which are necessary as catalysts for certain chemical reactions in the body.

SOURCES OF FIBRE per 3.5-ounce (100g) serving

Grains		Legumes		Dried oleaginous fruits	
Bran	40g	Dried beans	25g	Dried coconut	24g
Multi-grain bread	13g	Split peas	23g	Dried figs	18g
Whole wheat flour	9g	Lentils	12g	Almonds	14g
Brown rice	5g	Chickpeas	2g	Raisins	7g
White rice	1g			Dates	9g
White bread	2,5g			Peanuts	8g
Green vegetables		**Other vegetables**		**Fresh fruits**	
Cooked peas	12g	Cabbage	4g	Raspberries	8g
Parsley	19g	Radishes	3g	Pears in skin	3g
Cooked spinach	7g	Mushrooms	2,54g	Apples in skin	3g
Romaine	5g	Carrots	2g	Strawberries	3g
Artichokes	4g	Lettuce	2g	Peaches	2g
Leeks	4g				

For the past few decades, fibre consumption in industrialized societies has decreased significantly due to changes in diet.

The French currently consume less than 20g of fibre per day (Americans less than 10g) even though the recommended amount is between 30 and 40g. In 1925, the French consumed 7.3kg (about 16lb.) of dried beans (particularly rich in fibre) per capita per year. Today, they consume no more than 1.3kg (less than 3lb.), that is, five times less. Pasta has always been the staple of the Italian diet. Thirty years ago, Italians ate vegetables (rich in fibre) and high-fibre, whole-wheat pasta. Today, meat has replaced legumes and vegetables. Also, pasta is made with low-fibre, white flour.

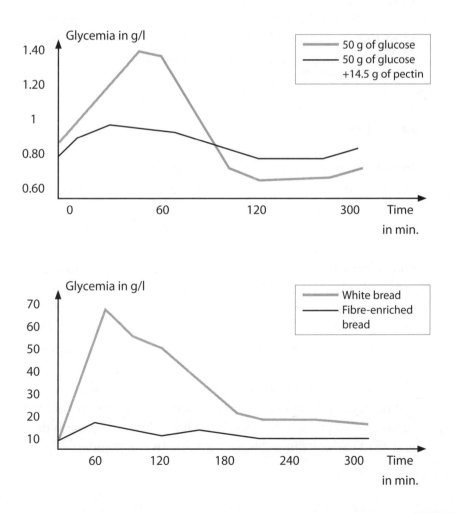

All of these changes have contributed to what medical authorities now believe has caused the rise in obesity and the alarming proliferation of digestive cancers[3]. It has been shown that fibre has an indirect beneficial effect on obesity. Its introduction into the diet can lower glycemia as well as insulinemia (the level of insulin in the blood), which is, as we will see in the following chapter, responsible for the storage of excess fats. The diagrams show that the presence of fibre in carbohydrates with a high GI leads to a reduction in glycemia and insulinemia.

SUMMARY

Proteins are substances found in many foods of animal and vegetable origin, namely meat, fish, eggs, dairy products (even skim), legumes, unrefined foods, and certain soy products. They are necessary for the body and do not causes weight gain.

Carbohydrates are substances that are metabolized into glucose, namely sweet foods (fruit, honey) and starchy foods (legumes, flour, roots, tubers, and grains). All carbohydrates are absorbed (when ingested on an empty stomach) in the same amount of time. This is why the old classification of carbohydrates into "slow" sugars and "quick" sugars is erroneous. They should be classified based on their glycemic potential, measured by the glycemic index. We can therefore make the distinction between "good carbohydrates" having a low glycemic index, and "bad carbohydrates" having a high glycemic index.

Lipids come from both plants and animals, such as in meat, fish, dairy products, and oils (olive, sunflower, walnut, etc.). Some fatty acids cause a rise in cholesterol (meat, whole milk products, palm oil), while others lower cholesterol (olive oil, fruits, fish fats and chocolate).

Fibre is a non-energy producing substance contained in foods having a low glycemic index, such as green vegetables (lettuce, endives, leeks, spinach, green beans, etc.) and certain dried beans, fruits and whole grains. Fibre-rich foods should be consumed in large quantities because of their nutritional value and their contribution to weight loss.

---

[3] See the publications of Professor Giacosa, Chief of Nutrition Services at the National Centre of Research on Gene Cancer.

CHAPTER 3:
WHY DO WE GAIN WEIGHT?

In Chapter 1, I explained the erroneous thinking behind calorie counting and weight gain. Nutritionists and other dietitians still think that the human body functions like a simple furnace: food produces a fuel known as calories, and the body burns this fuel as needed. Therefore, people gain weight because they eat more than they burn.

In this chapter you will learn why this thinking is false. More importantly, you will come to understand that extra pounds are essentially the result of abnormally stored energy caused by poor choices of food. You will begin to understand that it is the quality not the quantity of food that causes weight gain. In other words, people gain weight not necessarily because they eat too much, but because of what they eat.

THE ROAD TO HYPERINSULINISM

Since 1979, some nutrition researchers have clearly demonstrated the metabolic process behind weight gain. They concluded that "hyperinsulinism is present in all cases of obesity, no matter what the species or mechanism[4]." All the studies show that this hyperinsulinism is evident in where the weight is gained: above or below the waistline. For example, hyperinsulinism has a greater effect on androgynous obesity (situated above the belt, also known as the apple shape) than on gynecoid obesity (in the bottom half of the body, also known as the pear shape).

This means that someone who is only 10 to 20 pounds (4,5kg to 9kg) overweight has moderate hyperinsulinism, and that someone who is obese has high hyperinsulinism. We can logically conclude, then, that the real difference between an average weight person and an overweight person is that the one with the excess pounds produces high levels of insulin and that the average person does not.

Let us imagine that two people live together and eat exactly the same thing (and the same number of calories) every day. If after several years, one is overweight and the other is not, there would seem to be no clear explanation, except that the one who is overweight suffers from hyperinsulinism and the other does not. To understand hyperinsulinism, you must know about insulin.

In the last chapter, you learned the definition of glycemia: the level of glucose (sugar) in the blood. The normal level of glycemia on an empty stomach is about one gram per one litre (one quart) of blood. We also saw that as this level decreases (hypoglycemia), the pancreas secretes glucagon, whose role is to release a new supply of glucose into the blood. Glucagon, therefore, raises the level of glycemia.

But when the level of glycemia goes up (hyperglycemia), which happens after eating a meal, especially a meal containing carbo-hydrates, the pancreas secretes another hormone, insulin, whose role is to lower glycemia. So the amount of insulin needed to bring glycemia back to normal is proportional to the level of glycemia present. In other words, if glycemia is low, the secretion of insulin will be low. If glycemia is very high, the secretion of insulin will be high.

This is exactly what happens in a thin person. The amount of insulin secreted by the pancreas is always exactly proportional to the level of glycemia. On the other hand, for those who are overweight and especially for obese people, things happen differently.

In overweight people, as soon as the glycemic peak is attained, the pancreas begins to secrete insulin. But instead of releasing it into the blood in the exact quantity necessary to bring glycemia to its normal level, it will secrete an excess. Hyperinsulinism is caused by a pancreas that works overtime, and in turn, causes fats to be stored.

---

[4] Jean Renaud, Insulin and Obesity, Diabetologia, 1979, 17, 133-138.

When hyperinsulinism is not present, the energy of the meal is burned instead of being stored, and stored fats are released, allowing them to be used beneficially by the body. This is why we say that a thin person "burns" all the calories he or she consumes, especially fat calories. On the other hand, an obese person has a greater tendency to store fats and excess glucose than a thin person because of hyperinsulinism and insulinoresistance as well[5].

Hyperinsulinism is, therefore, if not a disease, at least a metabolic problem. The overweight and obese are individuals whose pancreases are more or less dysfunctional. When this was discovered at the beginning of the 1980s, researchers thought (and most still think) that if someone was hyperinsulinic it was due to heredity. Because those same researchers had noticed that hyperinsulinism disappeared when the patient lost weight, the only concrete advice they gave to overweight or obese people was to shed the pounds.

This led people to conclude that hyperinsulinism was the consequence of being overweight, which was the result of eating too much and not using calories efficiently. The conclusion for all of these specialists was simple as well as simplistic: "the only way to get rid of hyperinsulinism is to lose weight and to lose weight one must reduce the overall intake of calories and increase physical activity[6].

---

[5] For the obese person, hyperinsulinism is worsened by the phenomenon of insulinoresistance. In reaction to hyperglycemia, the pancreas secretes a large amount of insulin. Then, this quantity of insulin is not only excessive, but also poorly recognized by the body, without a doubt because the sensitivity of the receptors is defective. As hyperglycemia persists abnormally, the pancreas has a tendency to get out of control and then secrete a

THE OTHER HYPOTHESIS

Using this new classification of carbohydrates based on their glycemic index, I was attacking the problem from a different point of view. Contrary to those who had concluded that hyperinsulinism was caused by obesity, I formulated the hypothesis that obesity was caused by hyperinsulinism. In other words, hyperinsulinism was the cause and not the consequence of weight gain.

If, as I had observed, consuming carbohydrates with a low glycemic index stopped weight gain (and even triggered weight loss), it must be that it diminished (even stopped) its cause: hyperinsulinism.

The hypothesis that could be made from this observation was the following: obesity can only be the consequence of hyperinsulinism. But hyperinsulinism is itself, the consequence of high hyperglycemia. And high hyperglycemia is itself, the consequence of an excessive consumption of carbohydrates with a high GI. In other words, the consumption of carbohydrates with a high GI is indirectly (via hyperglycemia and hyperinsulinism) responsible for weight gain by favouring the storage of lipids as well as excess glucose, which is transformed into fat. Hyperinsulinism, in some ways, is the "catalyst" of obesity. To avoid and even halt weight gain, it was necessary to formulate a diet of carbohydrates low on the GI.

---

new dose of insulin, which only worsens the hyperinsulinism. It therefore creates a vicious circle for itself, in which hyperinsulinism supports insulinoresistance. Besides the excess storing of fats, insulinoresistance also poses an additional risk of a reactionary hypoglycemia.

[6] Dr. Jacques Fricker, Le métabolisme de l'obésité - La recherche, 1989, 20, 200-208.

GLYCEMIA LEVELS IN A MEAL

Since the 1980s, a large number of studies on diabetes has been done on GIs. Today, these studies provide us with a good understanding of the different metabolic phenomena caused by a variety of carbohydrates. Particularly, we know that the GI of a carbohydrate can vary based on several factors:

- The specific variety: Certain varieties of rice (especially Basmati) for example, can have a low index (50), while others (sticky rice) can have a high one (70).

- The method of cooking: Raw carrots have a low index (35) while cooked carrots reach 85. The index for potatoes grows according to the way in which the potatoes are cooked: 65 if they are cooked unpeeled in water, 70 if they are peeled before cooking, 90 if they are mashed, and 95 if they are baked or fried.

- Processing: Regular corn has an index of 70, but it reaches 85 when made into cornflakes or popcorn.

- Type of pasta: White pasta made under high extrusion pressure, like spaghetti, has a low GI (40 to 45 depending on the cooking), while ravioli and macaroni, which are not extruded, have a high index (70).

- The fibre and protein content: Lentils, which contain fibre (especially soluble) and protein, have a very low GI (22 to 30), compared to other starchy foods such as potatoes. In the same way, soy, which contains a high level of protein, has a very low GI.

Meals usually encompass elements from the various food groups. Some foods can raise the level of glycemia, while others help to moderate it. The important factor is the level of glycemia the meal produces. This is what will determine the final level of hyperglycemia and indirectly (if it is high) hyperinsulinism, which causes the abnormal storage of fats.

OUR SOCIETY'S DIETARY TRENDS

In the preceding paragraphs, I explained that the original cause of weight gain is the ingestion of carbohydrates containing a high GI, which causes abnormal storage of fats. But we can legitimately ask ourselves how some people who eat carbohydrates with high glycemic indexes every day can stay relatively thin. The answer is simple. It is because their pancreas, which is still in good shape, does not yet suffer from hyperinsulinism. But can a person stay thin all his or her life even though he or she eats a hyperglycemic diet? In effect, it is possible but less and less probable. Here is the reason:

- Some people can, in effect, stay thin their whole lives even though they have poor eating habits. This means that when they were born they had a healthy pancreas and, despite high hyperglycemia, which they endure all their life by eating bad carbohydrates, their pancreas are resistant enough to avoid hyperinsulinism.

• Other people (most people) also start out with a healthy pancreas that allows them to stay thin for many years despite their poor eating habits. Then, around the age of 30 or 35, and especially after 40, they begin to gain weight. Some even become obese and diabetic in their late years.

• This means that their pancreas was able to resist hyperinsulinism for several decades but that, because of the stress put on the organ year after year to fight against permanent hyperglycemia, it finally gives up. It is similar to a car engine that breaks down after a lack of regular maintenance. And then there are those (like me) who were born with an already unhealthy pancreas. This is why we logically attribute this deficiency to heredity. It is true that when one has obese parents (whose bodies produce too much insulin), there is a strong probability that his or her own pancreas will be fragile. It is inevitable in any case when the dietary habits developed at a young age are highly hyperglycemic.

In 1997, the World Health Organization denounced the world's obesity epidemic. Until that time, we thought that only Americans had a problem with excess weight. But now we know that it is an endemic problem in western countries, and it is slowly finding its way into developing countries as well.

Also in 1997, a large study showed that in the United States[7] obesity, paradoxically, has increased by 31 percent over the last 10 years, even though during the same period the average caloric intake had decreased, the consumption of fats had fallen by

11 percent and the number of people consuming low-fat products had risen to 76 from 19 percent. This survey showed that the cause of weight gain was separate from the amount of calories consumed because that amount had significantly decreased. Instead, I believe that the modern diet's low nutritional quality has caused this situation.

Looking closely at the glycemic index chart (p. 42), the high-glycemic foods in the left-hand column are foods that are refined (flour, sugar, white rice), processed (cornflakes, puffed rice, modified starches, chocolate bars) or "new" foods that have only been eaten regularly for fewer than two centuries (potatoes, white flour or, again, sugar). It is not difficult to see that all of these foods are precisely those consumed today in most Western countries and that, with worldwide spread, they are invading the eating habits of the rest of the world.

The low-glycemic carbohydrates listed in the right-hand column of the chart are, for the most part, foods most people don't eat (whole wheat bread, whole grains, unrefined flour, brown rice, etc.), foods that are rarely eaten (lentils, dried beans, split peas, chickpeas, etc.) or else foods that are not eaten frequently enough (fruits, green vegetables, etc.). These are all foods that were eaten in the past.

The diet of several decades ago was primarily composed of low-glycemic foods. Previous generations usually ate meals with a

---

7 F. Adrian, The American Paradox: Divergent Trends in Obesity and Fatintake Patterns, Am. J. Med., 1997, 102:259-264.

low glycemic count. Their pancreases were not over stimulated and as a result, the incidence of hyperinsulinism was low. At the beginning of the 20th century, very few people were overweight: less than three percent compared to up to 36 percent today for the USA's population and 14, 5% for the French one. What's more, only 10 to 20 percent of the population had a slight weight problem compared to 30 to 65 percent today, depending on the country.

On the contrary, our modern eating habits favour foods with a high GI. Today's meals produce a high glycemic count, which in turn over stimulates the pancreas to produce excess insulin or hyperinsulinism. According to a prospective study done in 1997, it is expected that a full 100 percent of the American population should be obese in 2039 if the trends of these last 30 years continue.

THE AMERICAN DIETARY MODEL

The United States unfortunately ranks as the most obese country in the world. By looking at the American diet, especially the fast-food trend, we can see why. Here is what Americans typically eat:

- Refined white flour (85): hamburger and hotdog rolls, sandwich bread, cookies and crackers
- Sugar (70), canned foods, sweet mustard, ketchup, crackers, cookies, ready-made meals, soft drinks, fruit juices, instant iced tea

- French fries (95)
- Corn consumed unrefined (70) or made into cornflakes or popcorn (85)
- White rice mass-produced (70) or made into rice cakes (85)

Americans are known for their high beer (110) and soft drinks (70) consumption and eat a lot of pre-cooked, processed foods, which all contain corn syrup (95), maltodextrins (95), and modified starches (95). The high-glycemic content, then, of the American diet can potentially lead to obesity, diabetes, and cardiovascular diseases. Unfortunately, these foods are more often consumed by the lower classes, and as a result, there is more obesity in their ranks. On the other hand, wealthier Americans are not as obese.

THE END OF THE FRENCH MODEL

Among western societies, the French exhibit the least amount of obesity. Even though there are more overweight people than ever before in France, they lag behind their Anglo-Saxon brethren.
The French diet is the reason. Unlike many countries, France, with its strong culinary traditions, has managed to resist the adoption of North American eating habits. But that resistance is waning among French youth. In the last 20 years, obesity has been increasing at an alarming rate. In two or three generations, the French population may be as hyperinsulinic and therefore obese as the Anglo-Saxons.

In conclusion, to answer the question I posed at the beginning of this chapter, we gain weight when we consume high-glycemic carbohydrates that force our bodies to store fat. And when we store fat, we gain extra pounds. In the following chapter you will learn how to shed your excess weight for good. This is the basic objective of the Montignac Method.

CHAPTER 4:
THE MONTIGNAC METHOD PHASE I WEIGHT LOSS

Now that you know that it is not how much you eat but what you eat that causes you to gain weight, let's discuss what those new food choices should be. In Phase I of the Montignac Method, you will learn how to modify your food choices to bring about the proper metabolic changes that we are looking for. In Phase II of the Method, you will learn how to maintain your ideal weight for the long term. (If you are at your ideal weight, you can proceed directly to Phase II.)

Since 1987, when I first came out with my Method, millions of people have successfully lost and maintained their weight. You can be sure to succeed, too, even if you have a lot of pounds to lose. If you are impatient to get rid of your excess weight for good, then I invite you to begin by applying the principles of Phase I, which is the actual weight-loss phase.

You will immediately begin to correct the dietary errors of the past and put your metabolism back in order.

The first thing you must do is calculate your goal weight. Use the information on body mass index (BMI) in Chapter 12 to do so. Take into consideration your sex, age, dietary history and heredity. These will determine how quickly you'll be able to meet your goal. At the beginning, it may be difficult to determine how many pounds you'll lose per week. Many report losing two pounds a week. Others lose less. Often, people will lose a lot at the beginning and slow down by the end. Just remember that each individual will experience weight loss differently. If it takes a little longer than your colleagues, do not be discouraged.

FOODS TO WATCH

Fundamentally, the goal of the Montignac Method is to lower the overall glycemic level of each meal while maintaining a balanced diet of proteins, lipids, and low-glycemic carbohydrates. But before you learn about making the correct choices, you need to know why it is important to watch out for certain carbohydrates.

Sugar

This is one of the worst of "bad carbohydrates." All food products should carry a warning about sugar's potential deleterious effects. Too many of us—especially children— eat far too much sugar. If I do anything with this book, I hope I can convince you how bad sugar is for you. Sugar not only causes weight gain, but also fatigue (see the chapter on glycemia), diabetes, dental cavities, and heart disease.

It's gotten to the point where we believe that we have to have sugar in our diet. It was only at the beginning of the 19th century that people even had access to sugar; it was considered a luxury. Today, I believe that sugar wreaks more havoc on our health than alcohol and drugs combined. You may be wondering what would happen if you cut sugar out of your diet completely. That's a good question. The body needs glucose (which is a source of energy), but not sugar. Fruit, unrefined foods, legumes, and grains are excellent sources of glucose. If you lack carbohydrates while you're playing tennis, for example, your body will draw on stored fats. So it is not necessary to eat any sugar to keep going. I urge you to give up sugar. If you can't do that, then I advise you to slowly wean yourself from sugar by using real fructose[8].

Bread

I could have devoted a whole chapter on bread because it is a huge topic. There are whole-grain breads, and then there are poor-quality, refined white breads that are found in most of our bakeries and supermarkets.

White bread lacks essential nutrients and fibre. The best that can be said about white bread is that it provides energy in the

---

[8] See chapter 9 on sugar

form of starch. Otherwise, it is completely devoid of nutritional components necessary for normal metabolism. Because it is fibre-less, it can cause digestive problems and constipation. The whiter the bread, the higher the glycemic level.

Whole-grain breads[9] made the traditional way with organic, unrefined flour are much preferred because they contain natural fibre. This is why their glycemic index is low (45). As a result, they are less "fattening" because they cause only a small rise in glycemia.

But no matter how good whole-grain breads may be, they will be restricted to your breakfast meal only during Phase I. First, its GI, although low, is still too high and, second, because the more carbohydrates we have during a meal, even with a low GI, the greater the risk (in Phase I) of noticeably raising insulin production. If you already consume a significant amount of another starch such as kidney beans or split peas, then it is not a good idea to add bread to your meal. What' s more, only bread with 100 percent unrefined flour and coarse grains rates a 40 on the glycemic scale; this bread is often difficult to find. However, we are now producing an exceptional "Montignac integral bread" (IG= 34[10]) in France whose GI is the lowest in the world. This bread is available on the web site: www.montignac-shop.com

Starches

Starches are complex carbohydrates. Some, like lentils or peas, rate low on the GI and are, therefore, "good carbohydrates."

However, other carbohydrates, like potatoes, or sticky rice have a high GI rank and are therefore classified as a "bad carbohydrate." They will not be allowed during Phase I.

Potatoes

You may not know that the potato originally came from South America. It was only in the 1500s that explorers to the New World brought it back to Europe. Initially, the French rejected potatoes outright and fed it to their livestock instead. But it was readily accepted by Norway, Germany, and Ireland, among other countries. In 1789, only when Parmentier issued the Treatise on the Culture and Use of the Potato did the general French population begin to consume it.

Fundamentally, the potato is a nutritious food, rich in vitamins and minerals in its raw state. Humans, unfortunately, have difficulty digesting raw potatoes because, unlike livestock, humans do not manufacture the necessary enzymes. As a result, we must cook potatoes in order to digest them properly. But cooking potatoes breaks down their beneficial starches.

Over the last 25 years, studies have shown that potatoes have an elevated potential of producing hyperglycemia. The potato is one of the worst "bad carbohydrates" because the GI of even a boiled potato (without the skin) is 70, the equivalent of sugar.

---

[9] There are 90 mg of magnesium in whole wheat bread and only 25 mg in white bread, based on a quantity of 3 1/2 mg.

[10] GI scientifically calculated by an independent and registered laboratory.

Other methods of preparation can boost its rating even more: mashed potatoes 90; French fries or au gratin 95. But if it is boiled in its skin, the potato can rank as low as 65. That is how it was often eaten in the past, along with other vegetables, which also kept the meal's glycemic level low.

Today, however, we consume potatoes in their most hyperglycemic forms (fried or baked), and they are generally only accompanied by meat, which is a saturated fat. As a result, the hyperinsulinism caused by the potato leads to greater weight gain than even the fats alone eaten during the meal. That means no more meat and potatoes during Phase I.

By the time you reach your desired weight and begin Phase II, you may find that you will start to choose boiled potatoes in their jackets over French fries. But even if you do eat French fries from time to time, you will learn how to utilize what I call "exception management." Exception management will help you learn how to eat out and maintain your weight. Most menus feature meat with potatoes. Instead of accepting the set menu, you will learn to ask for fresh vegetables such as broccoli, cauliflower, or eggplant. And if that proves impossible, ask for a salad. This will become an ingrained habit, at home and at restaurants.

Carrots

Just like potatoes, the starch in carrots is altered during cooking. When boiled or baked, carrots turn into a "bad carbohydrate" reaching a GI of 85. But in their raw state, carrots rank a 35. So, it is best to eat fresh, raw carrots. Unlike potatoes, they are easily digested.

Rice

Rice from Asia, especially long-grain Basmati rice has an average GI (50). But rice that has been mass produced usually comes with its high-fibre content stripped. The more starch rice contains, the higher its GI. Instant rice and rice cakes measure a GI of 85. Cooking also raises the GI of rice. The longer rice is cooked and the more water it is cooked in, the higher its chances of gelatinizing, a process that causes a rise in GI. But if you cook it slowly in two parts water for one part rice, the GI will remain low. The best rice to eat is long-grain brown rice.

Corn

Corn is a grain that has been a staple of the native populations of North America for centuries. The early varieties of corn are high in soluble fibre and therefore rank a 35 on the GI. But once the Europeans came, they began to alter corn genetically to increase output to feed livestock. Consequently, the GI of corn began to rise over the centuries. Today, when corn is made into flakes or popcorn, it can reach a GI of up to 85. Modern agricultural practices have basically rendered corn inferior to its original state.

Pasta

Because pasta is made with white flour, you may be thinking that I will have to eliminate it from Phase I. Surprise! In fact, it is a perfectly acceptable choice and it will help you to lose weight. Let me explain. Good pasta is made with hard or durum semolina wheat, which is rich in protein and fibre, even if the flour is refined. Pasta, especially spaghetti, also undergoes a process in which the dough is pressed through a sieve-like instrument under high pressure. This process is called extrusion. It wraps the pasta with a protective film that prevents the gelatinization of starches during cooking, but only under one condition: that the cooking time is no more than five minutes, reaching what the Italians call "*al dente*."

Therefore, extruded durum semolina pasta cooked *al dente* has a low GI of 45. If it is cooked longer than that, the GI goes up to 55. Chilling pasta can also lower the GI by five points. However you must know that in France we are making "very low GI Montignac spaghettis" whose GI is only 10[11] , the lowest in the world (www.montignac-shop.com)

Unfortunately, non-extruded pasta made from soft wheat, such as macaroni, lasagna and ravioli, has a high GI. Therefore, you must remain vigilant when you buy pasta. Nor is fresh pasta a good choice either. It is made with a small, manual machine that cuts it into strips. This pasta is not extruded. Chinese and Japanese vermicelli, on the other hand, are made from extruded soy flour (mungo beans), which naturally has a low GI. They are also cooked quickly in a matter of a minute or less. So, if you're going to eat pasta, choose Chinese vermicelli or spaghetti, which is the thinnest possible pasta available. Cook it *al dente* and serve it with a variety of sauces from tomato to curry, or even in a cold salad as an appetizer or a main course meal.

Legumes

Legumes such as kidney beans, lentils, chickpeas, and split peas are an excellent source of protein. What's more, they rank low on the GI. Green lentils, for example, have a lower GI (22) than green beans. There is a lot of misunderstanding about legumes, however. I'll never forget the time when an overweight man erroneously told me that beans make you gain weight. That is what his wife said. Meanwhile, he was gorging on potatoes, which made his situation worse.

Fruit

In our culture, fruit has become a symbol of life and health. You should eat some fruit every day. But the way in which you will eat it with the Montignac Method will be very different from before in order to enjoy all the benefits without experiencing the drawbacks.

Fruit contains carbohydrates (glucose, saccharide and especially fructose), but also fibre, which lowers its GI, diminishing the absorption of sugars. Apples and pears are especially rich in

---

[11] GI scientifically calculated by an independent and registered laboratory.

pectin (soluble fibre). The energy from fruit is readily available to be used by muscles and, therefore, will not likely be stored as fat. I suggest that fresh fruit be eaten by itself, either some time after or before meals. The reason: to avoid bloating, especially among the elderly.

Here's the reason why: If eaten on an empty stomach, fruit is quickly digested and flows throw the intestinal track unimpeded. But when you eat fruit at the end of a meal, for example, then it sits on top of the meal, especially a meat meal, fermenting and causing gas.

The best time to eat fruit is on an empty stomach, in the morning, for example, before breakfast. But you should wait about 15 minutes before eating the rest of your breakfast. You could also eat an apple or pear in the afternoon or late at night before going to bed, that is, at least three hours after your last meal.

As with all rules, there are exceptions. Some fruit with low sugar concentrations do not ferment easily. These are: strawberries, raspberries, black currants, red currants and blackberries, all of which can be eaten after a meal without consequences. Cooked fruits can also be eaten at the end of meals because they do not ferment in the stomach.

You must not forget, however, that cooking destroys their supply of vitamin C. Lemon does not ferment either, so you can drink its juice (unsweetened) at any time or use it to flavour food (on fish or in salad dressings).

I strongly suggest that you eat fruit unpeeled, but washed thoroughly. Peelings are rich in fibre and vitamins and give the fruit a low GI.

Beverages

Among the important foods we still must discuss are beverages.

• Alcohol

Most of you have been told that alcohol makes you gain weight. Technically, this is true, especially if you consume large quantities. But there is a way to drink alcohol and not gain weight. On an empty stomach, alcohol is quickly and efficiently used up by the body, and as a result, it will not draw on stored fats for energy. Alcohol therefore halts weight loss. When the stomach is full, especially with lipids such as meat, fish, and cheese, alcohol metabolizes much more slowly and contributes little to the production of stored fats.

• Wine

During Phase I, you may have a small glass of wine (4½ ounces/130 ml) at the end of a meal. But if you are looking for results quickly, you may dispense with this amount altogether, especially if you're the type that can't have just one. But once you've reached your goal, you can have up to three glasses of wine daily without gaining weight. Wine is also good for your health. From the 1980s onward, study after study has

shown the benefits of wine, especially red wine. Medical researchers wanted to know why the rate of heart attacks was low in
France. When they found that the French drank 11 times more
wine than their American counterparts, wine was singled out as
the main reason. These studies led to the concept of the "French
Paradox," and that is even though the French diet is high in fat,
a known risk factor for heart disease, the rate of heart attacks in
France is three times lower than in the United States.

Studies in the mid-1990s finally tracked down the miraculous
property: antioxidants known as polyphenols. In moderation,
the polyphenols in wine may also prevent certain cancers and
even Alzheimer's disease. But if you wish to abstain from drinking wine in Phase I, you may find yourself in uncomfortable
situations when dining out. Here is what I suggest. If you can't
decline a glass of wine gracefully, go ahead and have some.
Instead of drinking it, however, just pretend to: wet your lips
instead. I personally practised this method for several weeks
and believe me, no one ever noticed that I was not drinking.
I do the same with bread. I'll take some, put it on the table, but
it just sits there, untouched, throughout the meal.

• Cocktails

I also advise you to avoid cocktails before dinner. Instead, choose tomato juice or mineral water with lime. The only acceptable
cocktail, in my opinion, is champagne or sparkling wine. Do not
drink it on an empty stomach. Eat appetizers such as cold cuts,
fish, and cheese. By doing so, the sphincter known as the pylorus

that sits between the stomach and intestine will close. That will slow down the absorption of alcohol into your bloodstream. Nevertheless, try to avoid before-dinner drinks during Phase I for best results.

• After-dinner drinks (digestives)

Forget about having a Cognac or other liqueurs after dinner. They are not helpful to weight loss. If you drink them to aid digestion, then you won't need them while you're on the Method, because it will help your digestion enormously, even after a big meal.

• Beer

Beer, in moderate quantities, is acceptable. But you already are familiar with the fact that beer can cause bloating, weight gain (especially if quaffed on an empty stomach), bad breath, and indigestion. Beer not only contains alcohol, but also maltose, a carbohydrate whose GI is very high (110).

The alcohol and sugar combination can cause hypoglycemia; fatigue and sluggishness (see Chapter 6 on hypoglycemia). So if you are a heavy beer drinker, drink less, especially between meals. During meals, you should drink no more than 250ml (8oz) maximum. But if you want to lose weight, it's best to avoid it completely.

• Coffee

Caffeine in coffee, tea, and cola drinks stimulates your digestive system and can cause a rise in insulin secretion, especially those who are highly hyperinsulinic. It is why I suggest that you try to wean yourself from it during Phase I. Start by drinking Arabica or decaffeinated coffee, which contains less caffeine. Then try to stop it altogether. If you are a heavy coffee drinker, it may be due to the fact that you crave its stimulating effects to keep you awake. Do you often feel sluggish around 11:00 in the morning or 3:00 in the afternoon? Then the culprit may be hypoglycemia (see Chapter 6). When you've reached your ideal weight, and your pancreas is functioning normally once again, you may allow yourself the odd cup of espresso after a good meal.

• Soft drinks

Carbonated drinks are nothing but a combination of synthetic fruit extracts and a lot of sugar (70). They are, therefore, banned during Phase I. Even if some sodas contain natural fruit extracts, they can still be toxic. For example, citrus-flavoured drinks have been known to contain significant amounts of hazardous substances like terpenes. In my opinion, the worst soft drinks are colas.

They should either be strictly prohibited or carry special warnings such as those found on cigarette packages: "This product is hazardous to your health." Dr. Emile-Gaston Peeters denounces the contents of colas. In an average size cola in Europe, he says, there is 21 mg of caffeine and 102mg of phosphoric acid. Caffeine has stimulating properties while phosphoric acid is intensely acidic and its high phosphorous concentration can upset the body's calcium/phosphorous ratio, which can lead to a serious calcium deficiency in bones. Says Dr. Peeters: "The conclusion is simple. Cola must be, in its present composition, formally discouraged for children and adolescents. It does not benefit anyone.»

So during Phase I, you should avoid soft drinks, especially colas.

• Milk

Whole milk is a complex food containing proteins, carbohydrates (lactose) and saturated fat. As we will see later, milk fat is bad (saturated). By drinking skim milk, you avoid consuming the "bad" fat.

Another way to drink milk is to use the powdered variety because you can use a lot of it to create a thicker liquid. Most of all, I recommend eating sugar free yogurts such as the plain or low-fat variety. Yogurt contains bacterial cultures that are beneficial to your health.

However one must know that although the GI of lactose is low (30), the whey fraction of the milk (called lactoserum) is highly insulinotropic. Therefore, milk and dairy product must be eaten with great moderation. No more than one yoghurt a day. On the contrary cheese is ok since there is no more lactoserum in it.

• Fruit juices

Freshly squeezed fruit juices may be rich in vitamins and minerals, but they are also devoid of fibre. As a result, they have a high GI. Commercial fruit juices often have sugar added and contain too much acid. Therefore, during Phase I, it's best to eschew fruit juices altogether, and eat whole fruits instead.

PUTTING PHASE I INTO PRACTICE: LOSING WEIGHT

Phase I is straightforward and easy to follow. However, you must understand the Method thoroughly before proceeding. And in order to do that, you are going to have to completely discard your ingrained notions about weight loss. All you really have to do is use your common sense.

That is: never skip a meal. In fact, you need to eat three square meals a day: a hearty breakfast, an average lunch, and a light dinner.

Phase I is based on two fundamental rules:

1. The food choices at each meal must be made in such a way as to control its glycemic reaction. When the glycemic reaction is low, insulin production is kept at a minimum, and fat storage will likely not occur[12]

---

[12] The fundamental principles of the Montignac Method were proven to work in epidemiological studies by Professor Walter C. Willett of the Harvard School of Public Health's Department of Nutrition in Boston, Mass.

2. There are two combinations of meals to choose from:

- **Protein-lipid:** Meat, fish, dairy or legumes combined with low GI carbohydrates (GI of 35 or less)

- **Carbs-protein:** It will thus contain no saturated fat and very few poly or mono-unsaturated fats. Carbohydrates with a GI of 50 or less.

BREAKFAST

Breakfast 1

Your morning meal will be a combination of few fats and low-GI carbohydrates. As soon as you wake up, have one or more pieces of fruit. Wait 15 minutes and then eat the rest of your meal.

First option: High-fibre bread (100 percent whole wheat or whole-grain breads with at least 8 to 10 grams of fibre). Health food stores and fine-food shops usually carry these wholegrain beads. A special line of my whole-grain breads is also available[13].

Read your labels carefully. Many bakeries claim that their breads are whole-wheat, but the percentage of white flour is often higher than the whole wheat flour. Watch out for added sugar and

[13] For more information on Michel Montignac's products, visit my website: www.montignac-shop.com

saturated fats like palm oil. On the other hand, real whole-grain bread is made with all the nutritious components of the wheat grain, which makes it a "good" carbohydrate with a low GI. It is also chock-full of protein, minerals, and B vitamins. Other choices include pumpernickel and whole-wheat crackers.

You can spread your bread or crackers with sugar-free marmalade or fat-free cottage cheese, plain yogurt, or soya yoghurt. You can also mix the marmalade into the cottage cheese or yogurt. Avoid butter, margarine, honey, apple syrup, and jams, which contain 65 percent sugar.

Second option: Unsweetened, whole-grain cereals such as oats or quinoa. Avoid cereals that contain sugar, honey, caramel, corn (cornflakes, GI 85), and puffed rice (GI 85). You can use skim milk or plain yogurt mixed with unsweetened marmalade. All high-fibre bran cereals can be used sparingly, sprinkling some on top of your yogurt, for example.

To recap Breakfast 1:

- fruit (eaten 15 minutes before)
- whole-grain bread or cereal
- skim milk or yogurt
- sugar-free marmalade (optional)

Breakfast 2

This meal will draw from the protein-lipid combination. It can include: ham, bacon, cheese, or eggs (scrambled, sofboiled or fried). No carbohydrates, no matter what their GI is, will be allowed. That's because we want to avoid increasing insulin levels causing the body to store fat. This breakfast is a good choice when you are travelling, or have to attend a business over breakfast. Hotels and restaurants don't normally offer unsweetened, high-fibre breads or cereals.

N.B.: Do not eat Breakfast 2 if you plan to exercise because it doesn't contain any carbohydrates, which are a necessary energy source for physical activity. Also, don't make this breakfast a habit. It is high in saturated fat, and it is not recommended for people with high cholesterol and/or cardiovascular problems. To balance this breakfast out with the rest of your meals for the day, make sure you choose a lunch or dinner rich in "good" carbohydrates and low in saturated or "bad" fat.

BREAKFAST BEVERAGES

Here is a list of acceptable beverages, regardless of which breakfast option you choose:

- decaffeinated coffee (or coffee containing little caffeine, such as Arabica)
- weak tea (you want to keep caffeine at a minimum)

- chicory (alone or with decaffeinated coffee)
- skim milk (the powdered form can provide a thicker, palatable mixture)
- almond or soy milk

During Phase I, chocolate-flavoured drinks like hot cocoa or chocolate milk should be avoided. (Children can drink a sugar-free, non-fat mix.). Sugar must not be added to any of these beverages. Artificial sweeteners like aspartame should be avoided. Ideally, though, you should learn to enjoy beverages without a sweet taste.

LUNCH

Your mid-day meal, whether at home or at a restaurant, should consist of proteins, lipids and low GI carbohydrates. Choose your proteins from the meat, fish, egg, or dairy food groups.

Lipids can be derived from the fats in the proteins or added to food such as olive oil. Choose your fats with cardiovascular risks in mind. In other words, choose lean meats and/or low-fat cheese.

Carbohydrates must come from the low-end of the GI, 35 or less. A GI chart appears on page 42.

SAMPLE LUNCH MENU

- raw vegetables or soup (hot or cold)
- fish, meat or poultry
- side dishes (carbohydrates with a GI less than or equal to 35)
- salad
- cheese or yogurt
- beverage: water or 4½ ounces (130ml) of red wine or 8 ounces (230ml) of beer, consumed at the end of the meal (optional)

Appetizers

All salads are allowed, as long as they don't contain "bad" carbohydrates: no potatoes, corn, cooked carrots, beets or croutons. Real bacon bits are allowed. Dressings can include olive or sunflower oil, Balsamic or red-wine vinegar, or lemon. Don't allow any exceptions to be made to your meals. If you've asked for no croutons, and they appear on your salad, don't accept it.

Once you allow these exceptions, they will interfere with your success. You have to be adamant or else your server will not take you seriously. If you have difficulty being assertive, simply say that you are allergic to them. They will listen to you then. It works every time. Restaurants do not want to be responsible for a medical emergency.

Acceptable salad contents include green beans, leeks, artichokes, cabbage, cauliflower, tomatoes, endives, asparagus, mushrooms, radishes, cheese, meats, or even lentils, chickpeas or dried beans. What's more, you can eat as much as you like. Eggs are allowed, and freshly made mayonnaise can be added[14] Because we are not concerned with calories here, mayonnaise and a little bit of light sour cream are acceptable. Eat them in normal amounts. Avoid them if you have high cholesterol. Another acceptable appetizer is fish or seafood: tuna, smoked salmon, sardines in oil, crab and prawns.

The main course

Choose from meat, poultry, eggs, or fish, accompanied by a vegetable.

• proteins

Although meat and poultry are acceptable, fish is preferable for two reasons. Studies have shown that their fats are excellent for heart health, and our bodies don't tend to store fish fats. Some studies even show that fish aids weight loss.

Preparation: Ask for grilled meat, poultry, or fish. That way you'll avoid the pitfalls of fried, battered food. Batter is usually made from refined flour, a bad carbohydrate. Frying oils are usually made from saturated fats and are difficult to digest.

---

[14] If the mayonnaise is commercially made, do not eat it if it contains sugar, glucose, or flour

Also avoid regular sauces because most of them contain white, refined flour. Dijon or other hot mustards are acceptable. Avoid most other mustards because they contain sugar.

• vegetables

Choose from a variety of fibre-rich vegetables such as tomatoes, zucchini, green beans, eggplant, cauliflower, and broccoli. Check the chart on page 2. Failing that, have a plain lettuce salad: green, red loose-leaf or romaine lettuce, endive, and dandelion leaves. Salads can be eaten as an appetizer, during the main course or after with cheese.

• cheese after dinner

Meals in France consist of several courses: an appetizer, the main course, salad, and cheese. So, cheese is an option for you, too, especially if you are still hungry after your main course. Any kind will do, although dairy products such as cottage cheese should be kept to a minimum. But please don't eat your cheese with bread or crackers. It must be eaten alone. Having it with a salad is a good way to enjoy it.

Cheese and other dairy products, however, can be difficult for some people to digest, especially the elderly and those who lack the enzyme to digest a milk sugar known as lactose. Although not an allergy, lactose-intolerance can cause fermentation and uncomfortable bloating.

Dessert

Most desserts are made with three major ingredients: white flour, sugar, and butter. As such, they should be avoided. But my desserts are made from fruit, eggs and fructose, a natural sugar with a low GI. Some of my recipes also include dark chocolate containing more than 70 percent cocoa, minus the sugar (allowed in Phase II). See my cookbooks.

Once in a while, in Phase I, you can indulge in a dessert after your meal, as long as the carbohydrates in your dessert are no higher than GI 35. Some desserts can be made with fructose as long as they do not need to be cooked for a long time, such as pudding or custard, for example. I prefer using fructose because it has the same consistency as sugar and tolerates heat better.

Beverages

Avoid all alcoholic beverages in Phase I unless you are able to limit yourself to a small glass of red wine (125ml or 4oz) or beer (250ml or 8oz) at the end of a meal (never on an empty stomach). It's better to choose water, weak tea, or herbal teas. Similarly, avoid cocktails. Have tomato juice or mineral water instead.

If an alcoholic beverage is foisted on you, pretend to drink it. Just wet your lips and find a convenient spot to put it down and leave it behind. Use your imagination, too. Try pouring it into the champagne bucket, out the window or into the lavatory sink. During your meals, sip your beverage slowly, or wait until the second half of the meal to drink it. This is to avoid diluting your gastric juices that aid proper digestion. Drink water between meals, at least one litre (two quarts).

EATING OUT / RECEPTIONS

The food served at receptions can be a problem: chips, pop-corn, sandwiches, and the like. But here's how to avoid eating these "bad" carbohydrates. If there are little finger sandwiches, all you have to do is dispense with the bread and eat what's inside: salami, ham, egg, etc. Or look for cheese, sausage, or cocktail weiners. Raw vegetables are also an option.

Another way to avoid gorging on bad carbohydrates is to eat something before you attend the reception: a hunk of cheese, a boiled egg, a piece of fruit.

Here's a little story to illustrate my point. In the mid-1800s, my great-great grand-parents had a large family of six children. Once a year, the whole family was invited to eat at the house of the president of the company my great-great grandfather worked for. I was told that my great-great grandmother made sure that the children ate a hearty soup before arriving at the president's home. Feeling full, the children never developed a taste for rich foods that, of course, they couldn't enjoy at home. What's more, my great-great grandparents gained a reputation for raising well-behaved children.

Dinner at a friend's home

Eating at your friends' home can be handled diplomatically. If they are good friends, call ahead to find out what they're serving. Don't be shy about offering suggestions.

If your hosts are strangers, you will have to improvise. At every course, choose carefully. If a *pâté* is served as an appetizer, eat it without the cracker. If a cheese *soufflé* is the *entree*, have one serving only. (*Soufflés* are made with flour, so keep it to a minimum.) Take a pass on the potatoes and bread, but take as many vegetables as you wish: broccoli, mushrooms, green beans, etc. Cheese after the meal, as we have said, is acceptable.

When it comes to desserts, you may have some difficulty turning your hostess down. Insist on a small piece, and leave a good portion of it on your plate. Last but not least, wait until the second half of your meal to drink your wine. But only one glass. Even with the best strategy, it may be difficult to avoid eating bad carbohydrates at receptions or at dinner parties. Don't worry. Just compensate the rest of the day by rigorously adhering to Phase I.

The goal is to give your metabolism a rest, especially your pancreas, by keeping insulin production at a minimum. If you dump a lot of bad carbohydrates into your system, you may end up where you started. But look at it this way: you may have lost the battle, but you can still win the war.

DINNER

Your evening meal should be light, limiting your intake of fats, which when eaten at night end up in storage because of nocturnal hormonal activity and an inactive nervous system.

Dinner 1 (Protein-lipid type)

Start with a salad of raw vegetables, or a soup containing only "good carbohydrates." Then proceed with light proteins such as poultry, fish, cheese, or eggs accompanied by a low GI vegetable. Soups can be made with leeks, celery, cabbage, or other low GI vegetables. Remember, do not use potatoes.

To add some substance to the soup, stir in an egg yolk or puréed mushrooms. Keep your vegetables chunky. Large pieces in soups help with weight loss. Avoid soup bases because they are often made with sugar and flour. Some fish choices include mackerel and sardines.

Treat yourself to vegetables that are special, like an artichoke, which is rich in minerals, vitamins, and fibre. Steamed vegetables are best.

Dinner 2 (Carbs-protein type)

This menu will achieve the best results when it comes to weight loss. Like breakfast, it is composed of low GI carbohydrates, protein, and very little fat.

- vegetable soup
- brown rice with tomato sauce
- durum semolina spaghetti cooked *al dente* with tomato sauce
- lentils with onions
- whole-wheat semolina and vegetables
- artichokes with an olive-oil vinaigrette

Dessert can feature low fat cottage cheese or plain yogurt mixed with sugar-free marmalade. Cooked apples, pears, apricots, peaches or prunes in a compote also make for a lovely dessert. (When fruit is cooked, it doesn't ferment and cause bloating.)
Choose Dinner 2 as many times as you can every week. It's the best choice to get your eating habits under control with good carbohydrates, especially the legumes such as lentils, beans and chickpeas, which contain vegetable proteins. To make sure you keep some variety in your diet, here is how to set up your weekly menu:

- Fish: 3 to 4 times a week

- Meat: 3 times a week

- Poultry: 3 times a week

- Good carbohydrates: as side dishes at lunch and dinner and as whole-grain foods 3 to 4 times per week

- Starches with low GIs: Lentils, beans, peas, pasta, and brown rice should be included in most meals.

FAST FOOD

Deli sandwiches and food-chain hamburgers are probably the worst offenders of the Montignac Method. They all rate very high on the GI. But fast food is a reality in today's society. Unfortunately,nutritious fast food rarely exists. But if you're desperate for fast food, why not try a Montignac sandwich? Choose high-fibre, whole grain bread. (Toasting bread reduces its GI.)

Fill the bread with a low GI carbohydrate or lean poultry such as chicken or turkey. Your lunch bag or cooler can also contain your meal-on the go: a chicken breast, tuna, raw vegetables, or even a lentil salad.

INGREDIENTS FOR A MONTIGNAC SANDWICH ON WHOLE-GRAIN BREAD

Puréed green lentils	Dijon mustard	Herring
Puréed chickpeas	Fat free cheese	Smoked Salmon
Raw carrots	Fat free cottage cheese	Tuna in water
Tomato	Plain or fat-free yogurt	Turkey breast
Mushrooms		Chicken breast
Onion		Cooked ham
Green pepper		
Lettuce		
Artichokes		
Cucumber		

Believe it or not, you can also pop into your local convenience store and grab:

- Sliced ham (cooked or smoked)
- Hard-boiled eggs
- Tomatoes
- Cheese

Naturally, all of this should be eaten without bread. If your stomach is completely empty, have an apple or pear, apricots or figs. Eat as many as you like.

Because fruit is quickly digested, sometimes you feel empty soon after. Add a soy yogurt or nuts such as almonds, hazelnuts, or walnuts.

SNACKS

Normally, if you follow the Method closely and eat a filling lunch, you won't need a snack. But if at the end of the day, you get a hunger pang, it's best to fill up on something good. Avoid chips, popcorn, or pseudo-chocolate bars.

Instead, choose fresh or dried fruit, cheese or a soy yogurt. Fifteen minutes before you exercise, you can eat fruit. Your muscles will use up the energy produced by the good carbohydrates.

A bonus

If, at this point, you regularly eat white bread, sugar, potatoes, and desserts, you will lose the most weight on the Montignac Method: up to 10 pounds (4,5kg) in the first month. Don't let that success go to your head, though. Above all, don't go back to your old eating habits, either. Because if you do, you will gain everything back. Weight fluctuations are bad for your health.

OTHER CONSIDERATIONS

After your initial success, weight loss will continue, as long as you continue to rigorously follow the Method. However, the pounds will likely come off more slowly. In fact, your body will find its own rhythm, and the amount you lose may be different than your friend's. Men lose weight more rapidly than women.

Certain medications can interfere with weight loss, too. Excess weight in men is almost exclusively due to hyperinsulinism, whereas women have to factor in the effects of their hormones.

As a result, some women will have a more difficult time losing weight. Four possible causes for slow weight loss among women have been identified:

- Stress, which stimulates insulin secretion
- Hormonal disturbances, especially during adolescence or menopause

- Thyroid problems, which are more and more common
- Some women's bodies resist weight loss because of excessive yo-yo dieting (see Appendix III for more details)

If you have high cholesterol, the Montignac Method can help control your problem. Low GI carbohydrates and the fats suggested in this book will lead to a return of normal cholesterol levels in the majority of cases. Low-fat meats, fatty fish (Omega 3), olive oil, fibre-rich breads and cereals, and high-fibre vegetables and fruits are the mainstay of the Montignac Method Medical specialists the world over support this food regimen. In fact, there are numerous studies that support this trend (see Chapter 8 on hypercholesterolemia).

However, your doctor may not be aware of this new approach to food because it does not correspond with what he or she learned in medical school. The Montignac Method is a new approach to weight management and as such is going to take a while to catch on.

If your doctor questions your choice, you can assure him or her that you are eating natural, unrefined, fibre-rich foods full of nutrients.

You may even encounter some resistance from your friends or colleagues. The proof will be in the pudding. They'll watch as you lose weight, feel better, and look great. Not only will you lose weight, but you will also improve your metabolism and digestion. Your insulin levels will also be low.

TROUBLE SHOOTING

If you follow Phase I rigorously, you will lose weight. If your results are taking an unusual amount of time, something is not being done properly (see Appendix III). I recommend that you keep a detailed diary of everything you eat from morning to night.

Your diary will tell you what you are doing right and wrong. You could, for example, be eating too much yogurt and dairy products, or even regularly eating soup that you have been told only contains "good carbohydrates" when in fact it doesn't. Check the label. Even if the Montignac Method is easy to follow, you must, during Phase I, be motivated and make an extra effort to make it work. Do not compromise.

Some of you who have recently been on low-calorie diets should slowly change over to the Montignac Method. Your body may be too used to working with low-food intakes and if you increase the amount of food you eat, your body may initially end up storing it as fat. You may see a slight weight gain of five pounds before you start to lose them again.

To avoid that cycle, increase quantities bit by bit, day by day until you feel satisfied. If you've just finished a low-calorie diet, or if your diet was poorly balanced, you may notice at the beginning of the Method that your weight will stabilize even though your body is getting thinner. You may feel that you are losing weight, but the scale is not registering it.

The reason: you are regaining your muscle mass. The fat is being replaced by muscle. Although muscle takes up less room, it weighs more. If you're not used to a high-fibre diet, take it slowly at first. Add it day by day, not all at once. Otherwise you'll feel bloated and may have some abdominal pain and/or loose stools.

HOW LONG SHOULD I STAY ON PHASE I?

It depends on you and your individual situation. After you have calculated your ideal weight using the information in Chapter 12, you should continue with Phase I until you've reached your goal. Remember, each person will lose weight according to his or her body type and rhythm. Ideal weight varies. If you're feeling fit, then you can proceed to Phase II. If you feel you're at a balanced weight, then again you can go to Phase II. Similarly, if after a few weeks, your weight won't budge, then that may be the weight your body is going to remain at, and that will be your ideal weight.

Phase I could last several months if you have, say, 30 pounds (14kg) to lose. On the other hand, if you only have 10 or 12 pounds (4,5 to 5,5kg) to lose, then you can stop as soon as you have shed those pounds. Be mindful that Phase I also helps to retune your body and normalize your metabolism. It does that by re-balancing your pancreas in order to allow it to raise its threshold of glucose tolerance. This takes at least two to three months.

If you stop Phase I prematurely, even if you have reached your ideal weight, your pancreas may not have had enough time to return to its normal, healthy state. But if you continue in Phase I, you will feel physically and mentally more fit. Ideally, you won't even think about how long you should stay in Phase I because you will feel so good. In fact, the transition won't happen overnight. You'll want to make the move slowly but surely. It will not happen overnight, but rather quite progressively.

THE MAIN PRINCIPLES OF PHASE I

• Eat until you are reasonably full, without limiting the amounts that you eat or counting calories. But do not overeat.

• Eat three meals a day at specific times, and never skip a meal.

• Avoid eating between meals. Occasionally a snack is acceptable in the late afternoon; as long as it helps you eat a lighter dinner.

• Your menu should be varied, incorporating meat, poultry, fish, dairy, legumes, and a wide array of vegetables and fruit.

• Make sure your food is balanced by incorporating all three fundamental nutrients: proteins, lipids, and carbohydrates on a daily basis. Every meal must have at least some carbohydrates and proteins.

- **Breakfast** should include good carbohydrates and no fat.

- **Lunch** should consist of proteins, good fats and very low GI 35 or less.

- **Dinner** can be identical to lunch, but lighter and with few fats, composed of low GI carbohydrates 35 or less.

• Dinner may be composed only with carbohydrates (GI not higher than 50) but with no fat added otherwise the carbohydrates can be as high as GI 50.

• Limit your consumption of saturated fats (meat, fatty cold cuts, butter and whole dairy products), and instead opt for fish fats and olive or sunflower oil and skim-milk products.

• Avoid all sweetened beverages.

• Do not drink more than one glass of wine (125ml or 41/2oz.) or beer (250ml or 8oz.) at lunch or dinner.

• Drink weak or decaffeinated coffee and tea.

• Eat slowly in a relaxed atmosphere.

PHASE I: SUMMARY

In this chapter, you became familiar with good and bad carbo-hydrates. Good ones (low GI) help us lose weight; bad ones (high GI) cause a glycemic reaction and stimulate our pancreas to overproduce insulin. The key is to reduce the absorption of glucose. That depends on several factors:

- Fibre content

- Protein content

- Cooking time, which causes the gelatinization of starch. For example, when lentils are overcooked, their normal GI of 22 to 30 skyrockets to as high as 70.

- Industrial processing. Refined flour, for example, has a high GI and causes the body's insulin response to reach excessive levels. The excess insulin then causes the body to store the fats contained in the meal.

The glycemic index is the foundation of the Montignac Method. Weight gain, especially obesity, is caused by hyperinsulinism. And if someone is hyperinsulinic, it is because their meals are too glycemic.

Carbohydrates with high GI levels are the main culprit. Simi-larly, there are good and bad fats. Some raise cholesterol levels, others lower it. I explained that for more than 50 years, doctors, nutritionists, and dieticians have been on the wrong path.

They have been stressing the need to count calories and boost energy output through exercise. I, on the other hand, say that it is not the quantity of food we eat that makes us gain weight, but the quality of food.

Last but not least, the Montignac Method holds out the promise of returning your body back to its normal functioning health. Never again will you need to count calories or exercise excessively to no avail.

You can reverse your weight-loss failure, too. All this by eating normally, not restricting your amounts, and consuming healthier foods[15].

---

[15] For more information on studies of the Montignac Method, see Appendix V.

MENU SUGGESTIONS

PROTEIN-LIPID BREAKFAST

	Recommended	Acceptable	Prohibited
Fruit*		Apples Strawberries Raspberries Lemons Apricots	Preserves Canned fruit Fruit cocktail Bananas Chestnuts
Eggs		Eggs over-easy Soft-boiled eggs Omelette Scrambled eggs	
Fish	Smoked salmon Smoked trout Herring Shrimp		
Meat		Bacon Sausage Smoked ham Cooked ham	
Cheese		Fermented cheeses Fresh cheeses Plain yogurt	Hot dogs
Pastries Cereal Sweets Beverages		Only with fish : • Whole-wheat toast • Fibre-rich crackers Avoid bread when eating saturated fats: • Meats • Eggs • Cheese	All bread All cereals All pastries All cakes Sugar Honey Maple syrup
Drinks	Decaffeinated coffee Weak tea Hot chocolate (children only)	Skimmed milk	

*Fruit should be consumed on an empty stomach, 15 minutes before the rest of breakfast.

GOOD CARBOHYDRATE – PROTEIN RICH BREAKFAST

	Recommended	Acceptable	Prohibited
Fresh Fruit*	Apples, pears, orange, lemons, grapefruits, kiwis, peaches, grapes, nectarines, cherries, plums, strawberries, raspberries	Pineapple Papaya Mango	Bananas Chestnuts
Bread Pastries Cakes and sweets	Multi-grain bread Montignac integral bread, High fibre crackers (more than 20%)		White bread, Croissants, Pancakes, Danishes, Muffins, Biscuits, Waffles, Sugar, Honey, Maple syrup
Cereal and grains Yeast	Sugar-free whole- grain cereals, Oat bran, Wheat germ, Beer yeast	Whole-wheat bread Pumpernickel bread Rye bread Whole-wheat bagels	Sweet cereals Cornflakes Puffed rice Popcorn
Preserves	Sugar-free marmalade Sugar-free applesauce	Sugar-free granola Oatmeal Wheat bran	Preserves Jellies Sweetened peanut butter
Dairy and soy products	Fat-free or plain yogurt Fat-free cottage cheese Plain soy yogurt	Preserves made with fructose, Sugar-free peanut butter, Full-fat yogurt Low-fat cottage cheese	Sweetened full-fat yogurt Fruit yogurt Sweetened soy yogurt
Beverages	Decaffeinated coffee Weak tea Low-fat, sugar-free hot chocolate (children only) Soy milk	Skimmed milk Fresh fruit juice Vegetable juice	Sweetened fruit juice Soda, Cola, Alcohol Whole milk Chocolate milk mix

*Fruit should be consumed on an empty stomach, 15 minutes before the rest of breakfast.

PROTEIN-LIPID BREAKFAST MENUS

Breakfast #1	Breakfast #2	Breakfast #3
Fresh orange juice Apple	Fresh carrot juice Raspberries	Fresh apple juice Strawberries
Smoked salmon Multi-grain toast Tomatoes Cucumbers	Soft-boiled eggs Lean smoked ham Lettuce Tomato	Scrambled eggs Lean cooked ham Fermented cheese Mushrooms, Tomatoes
Weak coffee Soy milk	Weak tea Milk	Decaffeinated coffee Powdered skim milk

GOOD CARBOHYDRATE – PROTEIN RICH BREAKFAST

Breakfast #1	Breakfast #2	Breakfast #3
Fresh orange juice Peach	Fresh carrot juice Orange	Grapefruit/orange juice Kiwi
Multi-grain bread Sugar-free marmalade Fat-free yogurt	Oatmeal Preserves made with fructose Dried fruit Fat-free yogurt	Sugar-free granola Oat bran Wheat germ Fat-free cottage cheese
Decaffeinated coffee Powdered skim milk	Weak Tea Powdered skim milk	Weak coffee Powdered skim milk
Breakfast #4	**Breakfast #5**	**Breakfast #6**
Fresh apple juice Raspberries	Orange juice lemonade Pear	Apricot juice Prunes
Multi-grain bread Butter olive oil Fat-free yogurt Wheat germ	Whole-wheat toast Sugar-free applesauce Fat-free yogurt Beer yeast	Fibre-rich crackers* Sugar-free peanut butter Soy yogurt
Decaffeinated coffee Powdered skim milk	Decaffeinated coffee Powdered skim milk	Weak tea Powdered skim milk

* Crackers should be made without sugar or palm oil.

PROTEIN - LIPID BALANCED PHASE I MEALS (LUNCH OR DINNER) WITH VERY LOW GI CARBOHYDRATES

APPETIZERS

VEGGIES	FISH	MEAT*	OTHER
Recommended			
Artichokes	Anchovies	Cooked ham	Baked goat's cheese
Asparagus	Calamari	Dry sausage	Escargot
Avocado	Caviar	*Foie gras*	Fish soup
Broccoli	Cod liver	Salad with bacon bits	Frogs' legs
Cabbage	Crab	Salad with giblets	Hard-boiled eggs
Cauliflower Gherkins	Crayfish	Liver pâté	Mozzarella
Celery	Cuttlefish	Smoked ham	Omelette
Chickpeas	Herring		Sweetbreads
Cucumbers	Lobster		
Dandelion leaves	Mackerel		
Dried beans	Marinated salmon		
Endives	Sardines		
Green beans	Oysters		
Green peppers	Prawns		
Heart of palm	Scallops		
Leeks	Shellfish		
Lentils	Shrimp		
Lettuce (Romaine, red leaf)	Smoked salmon		
Mushrooms	Tuna		
Quinoa			
Radishes			
Raw carrots			
Soy germ			
Tomatoes			
Watercress			
Prohibited			
Beets		Terrines made with flour	Cheese fondue
Carrots (cooked)		White sausage	Croutons
Corn Rice			Dumplings/donuts
Pasta			Pancakes
Potatoes			Pizza
Tabbouleh			Puff pastries
			Quiche
			Soufflés
			Toast

*To prevent cardiovascular risk, choose meats with low saturated-fat content (see Chapter 8).

PROTEIN - LIPID BALANCED PHASE I MEALS (LUNCH OR DINNER) WITH VERY LOW GI CARBOHYDRATES

MAIN COURSE

FISH	MEAT*	POULTRY	OTHER MEATS
Recommended			
Bass Cod	Beef	Chicken	Andouilles
Herring	Lamb	Duck	Beef heart
Mackerel	Mutton	Goose	Black pudding
Red mullet	Pork	Guinea fowl	Ham
Salmon	Veal	Hen	Hare
Trout		Pheasant	Kidneys
Tuna Sardines		Pigeon	Venison
In general all salt and		Quail	Wild boar
freshwater fish		Turkey	
Prohibited		**To be avoided**	
Fried fish	Fatty cuts	Skin	Too-frequent consumption

*To prevent cardiovascular risk, choose meats with low saturated-fat content (see Chapter 8).

PROTEIN - LIPID BALANCED PHASE I MEALS (LUNCH OR DINNER) WITH VERY LOW GI CARBOHYDRATES

SIDE DISHES

Recommended			
Artichokes	Dried beans (white)	Leeks	Sorrel
Broccoli	Eggplant	Lentils	Spinach
Cabbage	Endives	Mushrooms	Split peas
Cauliflower	Green beans	Onions	Tomatoes
Celery	Green lettuce	Ratatouille	Zucchini
Chickpeas	Green peppers	Sauerkraut	
Prohibited			
Chestnuts	Couscous	Noodles (macaroni)	Rutabaga
Cooked broad beans	Gnocchi	Pasta	Squash
Cooked carrots	Lasagna	Ravioli	Turnips
Corn	Millet	Rice	

MISCELLANEOUS INGREDIENTS

CONDIMENTS, INGREDIENTS, SEASONINGS AND DIVERSE SPICES

To be consumed				Prohibited
Preferably in normal quantities			In reasonable quantities (not to be abused)	Caramel
				Corn starch
Baby onions	Gruyère	Anise	Bearnaise	Flour-based
Black olives	Lemon	Basil	Cream sauces	sauces
Celery salt	Parmesan	Bay leaves	Hollandaise	Industrial
Gherkins		Chives	Mayonnaise	mayonnaise
Green olives	Oils:	Cinnamon	Pepper	Ketchup
Homemade	• olive	Garlic	Salt	Maltodextrine
vinaigrette	• sunflower	Onion		Modified starches
Pickles	• peanut	Parsley		Palm oil
	• walnut	Shallots		Paraffin oil
	• hazelnut	Tarragon		Potato starch
	• grapeseed	Thyme		Sugar

EXAMPLES OF "BALANCED" PHASE I DINNERS WITH VERY LOW GI CARBOHYDRATES

Homemade lentil soup Over easy eggs Ratatouille Plain yogurt	Fish soup Cooked ham Green salad Raspberry
Split pea soup Stuffed tomatoes (see recipe in Appendix) Green salad Plain yogurt	Artichokes in vinaigrette Smoked salmon Green salad
Onion soup Tuna flan Green salad Cottage cheese	Leek soup Cold chicken breast, mayonnaise Green salad Baked apple
Endive salad Cucumbers in light sour cream Turkey breast Tomato sauce with basil Soy yogurt	Asparagus Poached filet of white fish Spinach Cheese

Beverage: water, weak tea, herbal tea, 125 mL (4.5 oz.) wine, or 250ml (8oz.) beer

PHASE I CARBOHYDRATE PROTEIN MEALS (DINNERS): FAT FREE*

Homemade vegetable soup Brown or wild rice with tomato sauce Sugar free apple sauce	Homemade vegetable soup Whole wheat spaghetti with tomato sauce Fat-free cottage cheese	Grated carrots Chickpeas with tomatoes Sugar-free applesauce
Lentils with onions (fat-free sour cream sauce) Green salad with lemon juice Low-fat yogurt	Baked tomatoes with parsley Dried beans (fat-free sour cream sauce) Soy yogurt	Mushroom soup Brown rice with tamarind Soy yogurt
Whole-wheat couscous with vegetables (GI<50) (without meat or oil) Fat-free sour cream sauce cumin + a pinch of bouillon	Cucumber salad Eggplant stuffed with mushroom purée and fat-free sour cream Dry plums	Lentil soup Quinoa with tomato sauce Baked apple

Beverage: water, weak tea, herbal tea, 125 mL (4.5 oz.) wine, or 250ml (8oz.) beer.
* Except a bit of olive oil.

PHASE I CARBOHYDRATE
PROTEIN MEALS (DINNER) : RICH IN FIBRE

	Appetizers	Main courses	Desserts
Choice of carbohydrates	Vegetable soup Cream of mushroom soup Lentil soup Tomato soup	Lentils Dried beans Peas Chickpeas Brown rice Whole wheat semolina *Al dente* spaghetti	Fat-free cottage cheese Fat free yogurt Sugar free apple sauce Stewed fruit Sugar-free marmalade
Recommandations	Without fats, potatoes or cooked carrots	Without fats (except olive oil and fish), served with to-mato sauce, mushroom sauce or vegetables	Sugar-free and fat-free

IMPORTANT INFORMATION ABOUT SALT

One may question about salt in only two cases: water retention and hypertension. But sodium is also involved in the intestinal glucose absorption. Therefore an over consumption of salt may amplify the carbohydrates absorption and increase the glycemia with the side effect which we know on the weight gain. Consequently, it is highly recommended to reduce the salt consumption if we really want to optimize the weigh loss process.

PHASE I MENUS "BALANCED" LUNCHES PROTEIN LIPID MEAL TYPE WITH VERY LOW GIs CARBS

Tomato salad Veal chop Green lentils Cheese	Cucumber salad Filet of cod (tomato sauce) Peas Yogurt
Radishes Turkey breast Puréed chickpeas Cheese	Quinoa taboulleh Filet of salmon Au gratin zucchini Cheese
Leeks in vinaigrette Grilled kidneys Cheese	Sardines in oil Spicy sausages Cabbage Cheese
Romaine lettuce Grilled game hen Broccoli Cheese	Smoked salmon Duck Mushrooms with parsley Mixed greens with cheese
Red cabbage Fish with capers Puréed green beans Cheese	Tomatoes and mozzarella Grilled chicken Green beans Cheese
Walnut endive salad Grilled ground beef patty Broccoli Soy yogurt	Hearts of palm Pork cutlets Puréed celery root Yogurt
Grated carrots Leg of lamb White beans Yogurt	Asparagus in vinaigrette Grilled black pudding Puréed cauliflower Yogurt
Meat bouillon with fat skimmed off Stew Leeks and cabbage Pears	Grated carrots Grilled salmon Spinach Apple
Tuna in olive oil Steak Mixed greens Baked fruits	Artichoke hearts in vinaigrette Rib steak Eggplant Soy yogurt

Beverage: water, weak tea, herbal tea, 125 ml (4.5 oz.) wine, or 250 ml (8oz.) beer

• To reiterate, in order to lose weight, each meal must not amount to more than 35 on the GI. This keeps the secretion of insulin to a minimum, which in turn inhibits lipogenesis, the storage process of fat. It will also stimulate lypolysis, the breakdown of stored fat, which makes you lose weight.

• This is the main goal of Phase I. By choosing low GI carbohydrates, and not worrying about calories, you will lose weight.

• Phase II will help you maintain your ideal weight. But, you could stay on Phase I for the rest of your life if you wish so. People who have done this have discovered a new vitality and well-being and don't want to stop.

• Even though Phase I is the basic nutritional reference, it excludes certain foods that are generally part of our normal diet, especially in social settings. Unlike low-calorie diets that make you feel deprived and creates a negative relationship with food, the Montignac Method actually helps you to enjoy food—maybe for the first time in your life. You may even become a gourmet cook. Eating, I believe, is one of the joys of life and gourmet cooking a veritable art just like music or painting.

• Cultivating the art of cooking makes you appreciate the vital necessity and the sensory pleasures of foods while creating dishes that please the palate.

• When I was a child, my parents often took me to the circus and the movies. Every time they took me out, I would get a chocolate ice cream for a treat. Of course, ice cream is primarily made of sugar and saturated fat. Consuming a dozen per year like I did at the time was not harmful. Today, in most homes, the freezers are full of ice cream. It is eaten practically every day.

• French fries are just as ubiquitous. In fast-food restaurants, they are served with almost every type of meal. Even if you ask to replace them with a salad, you get them anyway. That's how ingrained a habit French fries are.

• Occasionally eating an ice cream, a plate of French fries, or even a gourmet piece of pie won't hurt you. But if you eat those things every day, then it is no surprise that you'll likely gain weight. As Hippocrates so rightly said, "It is the amount and the frequency that make the poison."

CHAPTER 5:

THE MONTIGNAC METHOD PHASE II WEIGHT MAINTENANCE

Phase II takes the fundamental principles of Phase I and builds upon them. Remember, the goal of the Montignac Method is to keep meals low on the glycemic index. That way you won't stimulate your pancreas to produce an overabundance of insulin. If you've got too much insulin flowing in your bloodstream, your body responds by storing fat, causing weight gain.

So, you'll want to continue to eat low GI carbohydrates, low-fat meat and dairy products and fibre-rich foods. Phase II, however, offers you a little more leeway in what foods you can choose. Weight loss occurs when your meal total on the GI is no higher than 35. Weight maintenance occurs when your meal total on the GI scale is no higher than 50. But once you go over 50, you're at risk of gaining weight. Over 65 and you may be faced with serious weight gain, and possibly obesity. And it all comes down to what you eat. If you gorge yourself on the typical North American diet of French fries, donuts, cornflakes and white bread day after day, your likelihood of gaining and staying overweight is high. All of these foods hit the GI at 65 plus.

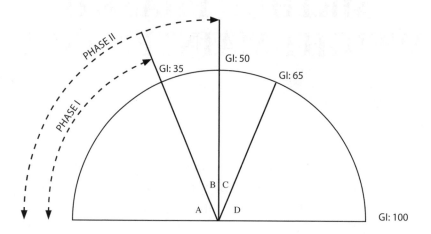

The Montignac method

This chart shows the glycemic index total of each meal required to lose, maintain, or gain weight.

ZONE A: GI of 35 or less = weight loss
ZONE B: GI of 50 or less = weight maintenance
ZONE C: GI of 50 to 65 = risk of weight gain
ZONE D: GI of 65 to 100 = risk of serious weight gain

Phase II is simply the second step to the Montignac Method. It is designed to help you maintain your ideal weight over the long term. You will be increasing the amount you're allowed on the GI. That's all there is to it. There's no returning to your old eating habits whatsoever. The Montignac Method is not a yo-yo diet. It is a new way of eating. It is a way in which you can consume food for the rest of your life. If you do start gaining weight and try to go back to Phase I to lose it again, your body will begin to resist your efforts.

The host of a famous French television program once confessed that he had tried my Method and found it to be very effective. But then he added: "The only bad thing about it is that as soon as you stop, you gain the weight back rapidly."
"Why didn't you follow Phase II?" I asked him.
Surprised, he told me he did not know what I was talking about. In fact, he had never read my book. He got his information from his friends and tried to apply it on his own.
Phase II can be followed two ways: with or without exceptions. In both cases, the goal is the same: to eat meals whose total GI doesn't exceed 50.

PHASE II WITHOUT EXCEPTIONS

This is basically Phase II with a broader scope. At its heart, you will be able to choose carbohydrates with a GI no higher than 50. Basmati rice (50) or *al dente* spaghetti (45) can be eaten with fish, for example. From time to time, you can also drink orange juice (40), eat kidney beans (40) or even sweet potatoes (50).

During meals, you get to boost your wine intake to two to three glasses or an entire bottle of beer, without jeopardizing your ideal weight. Your glycemia count, even if it increases slightly, is still low enough to keep any excessive insulin secretion in check.

You should still choose good fats (olive and fish oils) and limit your consumption of saturated fats, particularly in the evening.

PHASE II WITH EXCEPTIONS

This application of Phase II is a little more complicated and requires vigilance. It allows you to eat high GI carbohydrates under certain conditions. All you have to do is balance out the high GI with a food that will immediately lower it.

For example, if you want to eat potatoes, you'll need to eat them with their skins on accompanied by green lentils, a high-fibre, low GI carbohydrate.

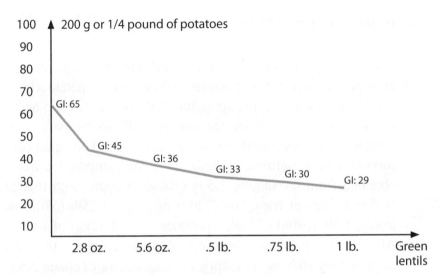

When you eat 200 g (1/4 lb) of boiled, peeled potatoes (GI: 65) with varying amounts of green lentils (GI: 22) you can lower the overall GI of your meal.

Eating potatoes with lentils is the way many people around the world eat their foods. By combining a high with a low GI carbohydrate, you bring the total GI down to an acceptable level. Take the Chinese diet, for example. They eat white rice, which is a high GI carbohydrate. But they always tend to eat their rice with plenty of low GI, high-fibre vegetables, which bring the overall GI count down to 50. In Phase II with exceptions, that is what you will have to do: combine high and low GI carbohydrates. Even though your calculations will not be precise, it will be close enough. But there is an additional piece of information that will help you decide on those combinations: pure carbohydrate content.

PURE CARBOHYDRATE CONTENT

Pure carbohydrates account for 55 percent of a baguette, for example; 33 percent of potatoes; 49 percent of potato chips; but 17 percent of lentils; six percent of cooked carrots; and a meagre five percent of lettuce and broccoli. To compare comparable things, the calculation of the GIs is based on equal pure carbohydrate quantities. Therefore, we can compare the index obtained from consuming 3.5oz (100g) of sugar with that of 10.5oz (330g) of fries, 7oz (220g) of chips, 1.25lb (570g) of lentils, 1.5lb (680g) of boiled potatoes or 4.5lb (2kg) of lettuce. All of these portions are comparable according to their GI because they all have something in common: they contain 3.5oz (100) of pure carbohydrates.

The goal of Phase II, then, is to manage the exceptions by not only knowing the GIs of foods, but also their pure carbohydrate content. To refresh your memory about GI values, refer to the chart on p. 38. So in Phase I, all you had to do was choose a carbohydrate with a GI of 35 or less from that list. In Phase II, you will still want to refer to the GI table as well as make some exceptions, such as the potatoes in their skins with some green lentils. However, you'll want to limit the occasions you do so as much as possible.

When you go to make an exception, you might reasonably think about choosing a low GI carbohydrate to compensate for it. Naturally you may think that the lower the GI, the greater the compensatory effect. You might also think that any green vegetable with a GI lower than 15 would be an ideal choice. In fact, you will be right as long as the pure carbohydrate content is the same. As we saw earlier, this concentration differs from carbohydrate to carbohydrate (see table on p. 42).

Traditionally, the carrot is considered to be in the same category as all other carbohydrates: potatoes or lentils, for example. But with my Method, this is not the case. You already know that cooked carrots have a higher GI content than lentils. Their pure-carbohydrate content is also different from this group. Indeed, there can be differences within the same family of carbohydrates. In the case of the potato, the GI changes if it is raw or cooked. We also know that the pure carbohydrate concentration also varies according to the same parameters. Cross-referencing the GI table with that of the pure-carbohydrate concentration, then, can reveal some surprises.

Among the good surprises are high GI cooked carrots. They actually rate low on their pure-carbohydrate concentration (6g per 3.5oz (100g), which is just a little higher than that of lettuce. We know, therefore, that when we choose to eat cooked carrots, we don't need to worry too much about exception management because cooked carrots have very little GI consequence, especially if you eat a small amount. On the other hand, compensating for the glycemic consequence of a baked potato requires eating four to five times more carrots, six times more to equal French fries. In other words, you would have to eat about 1.3lb (490g) of cooked carrots to induce the same critical result in glycemia as do 3.5 oz (100g) of fries.

The conclusion you may draw is that in Phase II you no longer have to be as obsessed with cooked carrots as you were in Phase I. If you come across a couple of slices of these colourful little carbohydrates, eat them without feeling guilty or even wondering how to compensate for them. The same process can be applied to all carbohydrates with a high GI whose concentration in pure carbohydrates is weak or very weak, especially turnip (3 percent), pumpkin (7 percent), watermelon (7 percent), cantaloupe (6 percent), and beets (7 percent). If you do not eat them often or in great quantity, they can help you to build up a certain tolerance.

There's some bad news, too, about high GI carbohydrates, which we will discuss in detail later. But right now, let's tackle French fries.

Frying potatoes not only boosts its GI to 95, one of the highest on the index, but it also causes the highest pure-carbohydrate concentration: 33g per 3.5oz (100g), 5.5 times that of cooked carrots, but also 3.5 times that of potatoes boiled, unpeeled. Potato chips outrank fries in their pure carbohydrate concentration with 49g per 3.5oz. of product with, I must note, a slightly inferior GI (80).

More bad news: sugar. Its GI is high (70), and its concentration of carbohydrates is the maximum (100 percent), that is, three times that of French fries and 16.6 times that of carrots. It would take 60 g of lentils to compensate for sugar to lower the resulting GI to 50.

The last bad surprise, of course, deals with white flour which, besides its high glycemic index (70 for a baguette, 85 for a hamburger bun), has a high pure-carbohydrate concentration (58 percent for very white sandwich bread, 55 percent for a baguette and 74 percent for refined semolina). This means that if you make an exception by eating white bread or anything else made with refined flour (pizza, pastries, cakes, pancakes, waffles, etc.) you will pay because if the quantities are substantial, you will have difficulty making up for it with good carbohydrates.

Let us look at an example that demonstrates how you can put this exception management into practice. Say you grab a white-bread sandwich at a bus station or a convenience store. The sandwich weighs about 7 oz (200g). To make up for the high GI of the sandwich (85), you'll have to eat 1.5 lb (700g). of lentils to lower your glycemic count to 53.

Of course, being at a bus station, you probably won't find a lentil anywhere in sight. So you may think that an apple might do to compensate. The only problem is that apples have a higher GI than lentils (33 instead of 22) and that they contain fewer pure carbohydrates (12g instead of 17g). This means that in order to bring the resulting glycemia down to 57 you would theoretically have to eat more than 2 lb (900g). of apples, which would be practically impossible.

Thankfully, there is a little trick you can employ: if you eat a low GI carbohydrate before a high one, the compensation phenomenon is much more effective. In other words, if you ate two to three apples first before your white-bread sandwich, the resulting glycemia count will be moderated.

So by eating your lentils, lettuce, chickpeas, spaghetti *al dente*, or fruit before your exception, the compensation will be more effective. One of the most important rules to apply in the management of Phase II is to anticipate the exception you will make. It is the only way to be prepared with the appropriate compensation.

It is Sunday in France. Unlike North America, the biggest meal is served at noon, not at night. Often, a beautiful pastry is served for dessert. In this instance, let's say it's a *tarte aux fraises* (strawberry pie). This pie not only contains both highly refined white flour (85) and sugar (70), but its pure carbohydrate concentration levels are 58 and 100 percent respectively. To compensate for this exception, the rest of your meal should consist of a low GI appetizer such as a plate of *crudités* with tomatoes, cucumbers, etc. or a green lentil salad. Vegetables for the main course should also be from the lower end of the GI scale, such as broccoli, cauliflower, green beans, etc. No bread, not even whole-grain, should be eaten at all, not even with your cheese course.

What's more, you can even indulge in your three glasses of wine if you wish, because the way you've set up the meal, your overall glycemia will be average, or at least sufficiently modest, to ensure that you will not experience excessive insulin secretion.

This exception management should not be abused. Don't expect to be able to eat a ton of lettuce to compensate for a bucket-full of French fries. It doesn't work that way. What you would be doing there is simply eating poorly. And that will guarantee a weight gain. Because too many carbohydrates, regardless of their GIs, will be transformed into fat.

The key is the pure-carbohydrate concentration. As we saw previously, even if the GI of cooked carrots and French fries is similar, the pure-carbohydrate concentration of the fries is eight times greater. That means that if you eat fries, your portion size must always remain modest. You obviously will have to apply the same rule to white flour and sugar which, as we saw before, are, along with fries and chips, the mega champions of bad carbohydrates because they have both a very high GI and a very high pure-carbohydrate concentration.

Another key is to anticipate your exceptions so that you can prepare for their compensations. Try to know beforehand what you will be eating from the beginning to the end. Otherwise, if you make a huge exception at the beginning of a meal, it may be too late to compensate for it. It is always best to know what is in store for you at the start of the meal so that you will be able to make the best choices.

For example, you can eat your exception at appetizer stage, say a puff pastry. During the main course, you can have an exception of a boiled potato as long as you have fish. You can have bread and compensate with cheese.

Don't try to make an exception twice in a row, like having puffed pastry for your appetizer and then mashed potatoes or polenta during your main course. By dessert, you'll try to compensate for those choices and you'll have to gorge on a ton of lettuce or lentils, which would be impossible. This would be a poor solution anyway because the amount of carbohydrates that all of that would represent would still raise your glycemia.

Phase II, then, would be best described as controlled freedom, whose fundamental principles must become second-nature to you. All exceptions are based on two notions: that they be exceptional and that they be well managed. Also, exceptions need to be made by calculating their GI as well as their pure-carbohydrate concentrations.

And if you do anything, try to choose your exceptions from those with weak, pure-carbohydrate concentrations. That way, they would be easy to compensate for. However, don't fool yourself into believing that there is a distinction between "small" and "big" exceptions, with the latter the only exception you make a compensation for.

In effect, you could consider drinking three glasses of wine with dinner or eating a small piece of white-bread toast small exceptions, since it is true that the negative effects of these on your weight are almost negligible.

But this attitude does not come without a price because you risk minimizing the so-called "small" exceptions by making them habits. And just as small streams make large rivers, several small exceptions for which you do not compensate during a meal can have the same unhealthy effects as the large exceptions.

By becoming less and less vigilant, you'll forget the fundamental principles of the Method. Always make yourself aware that you have made an exception, and quickly figure out what you'll do to rebalance your system. That's a fundamental principle of Phase II. Don't compromise and don't give in even in social situations.

Sure, you'll have a function in which they'll serve you mini-quiches, potatoes and a cake filled with flour, butter, and sugar. But you'll have to choose how to proceed. Don't get trapped into thinking you have no choice. You do. There is always something that you can do. Work from a place of strength. If you've successfully completed Phase I, you can take that success and build on it.

Take vegetarians, for example. By choosing not to eat meat, they are constantly faced with making decisions on what to have. Their conviction not to eat meat helps them to remain true to their commitment. Even when they are invited to a barbecue, they'll just eat the salad. If you've been served with potatoes, look for a salad or a bit of cheese. You could even eat the Black Forest cake dessert by discreetly nibbling on the parts that are acceptable, like the strawberries. Although you weren't able to make compensation, you didn't create a catastrophe either. But don't forget about this meal either.

Be vigilant during your next couple of meals and try to compensate with them, even eating Phase I meals for a while. No matter what happens, your scale will be your best feedback. If you gain some weight, here are two reasons that might apply: either your pancreas has not yet found its acceptable level of tolerance and is still very sensitive to even the slightest rise in glycemia, or the amount and frequency of your exceptions happen too often.

You should then take the necessary measures, doubling your attention and especially going back to Phase I as often as possible. But there will be another, more telling sign: the state of your health. If you go too far, you'll feel the awful effects. You may feel less energetic and experience more fatigue.
You will naturally go back to what feels best for you.

EXAMPLE OF EXCEPTION MANAGEMENT
(EXCEPTIONS ARE IN **BOLD** PRINT, COMPENSATORY)

lentil salad with olive oil vinaigrette veal chop **white rice** green salad yogurt	grated carrots cod green beans **crème brûlée**	**crème caramel** split pea soup cooked ham **mashed potatoes** **with olive oil** plain strawberries
al dente spaghetti salad **slice of pizza** green salad sugar-free apple sauce	caesar salad without croutons sausage puréed split peas vanilla bean ice cream	**cantaloupe** **buckwheat crepe with eggs** **and ham** green salad raspberries
smoked salmon green salad leg of lamb legumes cheese + 2 slices of bread	**foie gras on** **3 cocktail toasts** duck ratatouille green salad cheese	green salad chili con carne **plum pie**
leeks in vinaigrette lentils with ham **chocolate eclair**	**12 oysters and 2 slices** **of rye bread** marinated salmon green salad chocolate mousse cake made with 70% cocoa	artichoke hearts *al dente* spaghetti with cream of soy / or curry sauce **cheesecake**
al dente spaghetti pork chop green lentils cheese + **2 slices of bread**	vegetable soup leeks, cabbage, celery zucchini sorrel omelette green salad	watermelon rib steak broccoli fresh poached apricots in fructose

	AVERAGE PURE CARBOHYDRATE CONCENTRATION	GLYCEMIC INDEX	GLYCEMIC OUTCOME
Beer	5	110	5,5
Baked potatoes	25	95	23,75
French fries	33	95	31,35
Puffed rice	85	85	72,25
Instant rice	24	85	20,4
Cooked carrots	6	85	5,1
Corn-flakes	85	85	72,25
Plain Pop Corn (without sugar)	63	85	53,55
Flour T45 (white bread)	58	85	49,3
Tapioca	94	85	79,9
Turnips (cooked)	3	85	2,55
Corn starch	88	85	74,8
Mashed potatoes	14	80	11,2
Cooked broad beans	7	80	5,6
Crackers	60	80	48
Pumpkin/Squash	7	75	5,25
Watermelon	7	75	5,25
Rice cakes	24	70	16,8
Flour T55 (baguette)	55	70	38,5
Sweetened cereals	80	70	56
Boiled peeled potatoes	20	70	14
Sugar (saccharose)	100	70	70
Instant non sticky rice	24	70	16,8
Cola	11	70	7,7
Chocolate bars	60	70	42
Noddles, ravioli	23	70	16,1
Corn	22	65	14,3
Unpeeled boiled potatoes	14	65	9,1
Jam (regular)	70	65	45,5
Dried Raisins	66	65	42,9
Whole wheat bread (T150)	47	65	30,55
Refined semolina	25	65	16,25
Honey	80	60	48
Melon	6	60	3,6
Banana	20	60	12
Long grain white rice	23	60	13,8
Butter cookies	75	55	41,25
White pasta	23	55	12,65
Buckewheat pancake	25	50	12,5
Sweet potato	20	50	10
Basmati rice	23	50	11,5
Whole brown rice	23	50	11,5

Whole wheat pasta (T150)	19	50	9,5
Natural apple juice	17	50	8,5
Kiwi	12	45	5,4
Bran bread	40	45	18
Fresh wholewheat bread	45	45	20,25
Pumpernickel bread	45	45	20,25
Grapes	16	45	7,2
Sorbet	30	40	12
Buckewheat flour	65	40	26
al dente spaghetti	25	40	10
Wholewheat (100%) pasta (T200)	17	40	6,8
Fresh peas	10	35	3,5
Kidney beans	11	35	3,85
Ancestral Indian corn	21	35	7,35
Quinoa (cooked)	18	35	6,3
Dried peas (cooked)	18	35	6,3
Orange	9	35	3,15
Dried apricots	63	35	22,05
Peaches	9	35	3,15
White beans	17	35	5,95
Apple	12	35	4,2
Montignac integral bread	55	34	18,7
Chinese vermicelli (mungo)	15	30	4,5
Raw carrots	7	30	2,1
Pears, figs	12	30	3,6
Milk (2% fat)	5	30	1,5
Green beans	3	30	0,9
Brown lentils	17	30	5,1
Chickpeas (cooked)	22	30	6,6
Plums, grapefruits	10	30	3
Fresh apricots	10	30	3
Garlic	5	30	1,5
Dark chocolate (+ 70% de cacao)	17	25	4,25
Green lentils	17	25	4,25
Split peas	22	25	5,5
Cherries	17	25	4,25
Fructose	100	20	20
Soy (cooked)	15	20	3
Montignac sugar free jam	40	20	8
Peanuts	9	15	1,35
Walnuts	5	15	0,75
Onion	5	15	0,75
Montignac low GI spaghetti (GI = 10)	25	10	2,5
Green vegetables, (lettuce, mushroom, tomatoes, eggplant, green pepper, etc.)	5	10	0,5

CHAPTER 6:
HYPOGLYCEMIA: THE DISEASE OF THE CENTURY

When I talk about metabolism, I'm referring to the transformation of food into vital elements the body needs to function. The metabolism of lipids, for example, is the conversion of lipids into fats. This book's focus is primarily on the metabolism of carbohydrates and their consequences. As explained before, insulin, which is manufactured by the pancreas, plays an essential role in carbohydrate metabolism. Insulin acts upon blood glucose, easing its penetration into cells. It also assures the proper functioning of organs, aids in the formation of glycogen by the muscles and liver, and induces the synthesis of fat reserves. Insulin expels glucose (sugar) from the blood and, thus, lowers the glucose level in the blood (glycemia). If the amount of insulin is disproportionate to the glucose that it is meant to metabolize, then the blood glucose level falls to an abnormally low level. The body is then in a state of hypoglycemia.

Hypoglycemia, then, is not always caused by a glucose deficiency, but often by an excessive secretion of insulin (hyperinsulinism) following excess consumption of carbohydrates with high GIs such as potatoes, white bread, corn, and so forth.

You may be familiar with the mid-morning or mid afternoon slump. Even after a good night's sleep, you suddenly feel tired for no apparent reason. More than likely, though, your blood glucose level may be lower than normal. If that is the case, then you are experiencing hypoglycemia. If you try to boost your energy by eating a cookie or a candy (both bad carbohydrates with high GIs), your body will quickly metabolize it into glucose. The increase of glucose in the blood will make you feel better—temporarily.

But the presence of glucose in the blood will also automatically trigger the secretion of insulin, which will deplete your blood of glucose, returning you to a hypoglycemic state worse than before you ate your treat. It is this vicious circle that can lead to addictive sugar cravings.

Some scientists have seen a link between alcoholism and chronic hypoglycemia. When an addict's blood alcohol level begins to drop, he or she feels down and begins to crave another drink. Alcoholics are also known to consume carbohydrates with high GIs. The combination of high-GI carbohydrates and alcohol in the bloodstream increases the risk of hypoglycemia and its attendant fatigue. The alcoholic will try to compensate for this fatigue by taking another drink, inducing a state of transitional elation. What's worse is when the addict drinks alcoholic beverages that are sweet, such as rum and Coke, gin and tonic, screwdriver, sherry, and so forth. In this case, the risk of hypoglycemia increases exponentially.

Another population at risk are teenagers. Because they are huge consumers of sweet beverages like pop, they have a similar glycemic profile as that of the alcoholic. Some American doctors have contended that this phenomenon actually predisposes young people to alcoholism, which is reaching epidemic proportions on university campuses. Parents can protect their children by eliminating sugar and high-GI carbohydrate food such as pop, candies, popcorn, and potato chips, among other things, from their diets. The symptoms of hypoglycemia are:

- Fatigue, sudden exhaustion
- Nervousness
- Irritability
- Mood swings
- Impatience
- Anxiety
- Yawning, lack of concentration
- Headaches
- Excessive perspiration
- Sweaty palms
- Disorganized work or study habits
- Digestive problems
- Nausea
- Difficulty speaking

While this list is not exhaustive, it is significant. A person suffering from hypoglycemia won't necessarily exhibit all of these symptoms, nor are the symptoms permanent. Some symptoms such as nervousness, moodiness, and irritability can flare up right before meals and vanish once something has been eaten. But there is one symptom that is universal: fatigue.

Fatigue is one of the most common complaints of our time. It is ironic that the more people tend to sleep, have time for leisure, or go on vacation, the more tired they seem to be. When they get up in the morning, they feel tired. By the time lunch rolls around, they are exhausted. By mid-afternoon, they're napping at their desks.

When it's time to go home, they drag themselves to their cars and make the long commute home. In the evening, they fall asleep watching TV. Strangely enough, once they go to bed, they are no longer tired. But when they do finally fall asleep, it's often time to wake up and then the whole process starts all over again. They blame the reason for their fatigue on stress, noise, pollution and the frantic pace of their lives. They try to fight back by drinking coffee, eating sweets, taking vitamin and mineral supplements, exercising or doing yoga. But if they only ate differently, maybe things would change.

You see, I believe that the fundamental reason most people are tired is because they eat too many high-GI carbohydrates. The North American diet is packed with too many potatoes, sugar, white rice, cookies, popcorn, and sweet beverages, among other things. As a result, there's too much insulin and too little glucose floating around in the bloodstream, which causes hypoglycemia and fatigue.

Until recently, medical researchers believed that only overweight people were hypoglycemic. But studies conducted in the United States over the last 10 years have disproved this theory. Thin people can also suffer from hypoglycemia. The difference between them is metabolism. Some gain weight, while others do not. But as far as blood glucose is concerned, the phenomenon and its consequences are identical. These U.S. studies also reveal that women are more susceptible to glycemic fluctuations. This could explain the reason behind women's frequent mood swings. There even has been a strong association between postpartum depression and hypoglycemia.

On the Montignac Method, not only will you lose weight, but you'll also return to a healthy state of well-being. That's because low-GI carbohydrates do not cause hypoglycemia. Indeed, you'll feel more energetic, optimistic and enjoy life more. No longer will you experience chronic fatigue. When you eliminate sugar from your diet and limit your intake of bad carbohydrates, your pancreas will halt its excess secretion of insulin. As a result, your blood glucose level will return to normal.

According to the scientists and doctors with whom I work, hypoglycemia is one of the most difficult diseases to diagnose. The symptoms are so varied that family doctors rarely identify it. One way to know if you suffer from hypoglycemia is to practice the Montignac Method. After about a week on it, you will likely notice a sense of well-being.

Fatigue can also be caused by vitamin, mineral or other nutritional deficiencies. Those who follow low-calorie diets lack important nutrients because they do not eat enough. Over processing and poor agricultural practices also reduce the nutritional value of today's foods.

In order to stay healthy and avoid hypoglycemia, eat low GI carbohydrates, such as whole-grain products, legumes, vegetables, and fruits. Whenever you can, eat vegetables and fruits raw to derive the most nutrients as possible.

Your body will thank you for it.

CHAPTER 7:
VITAMINS, MINERALS AND TRACE ELEMENTS

There are many reasons that modern foods have been depleted of their essential vitamins, minerals and trace elements.
The main causes are: refining techniques, industrial processing,
and conservation. Cooking methods, too, cause food to lose its
nutritional value. Even though we've been aware of the poor
quality of our foods for some time now, it seems that nothing
is being done about it. The result is an increase in illness, especially fatigue and difficulty losing weight.

VITAMINS

In the word "vitamin" is vita, which is Latin for "life." The
metabolism of food would not be possible without vitamins.
These organic substances play an important role in the function

of hundreds of enzymes by triggering biochemical reactions within our body cells.

It seems ironic that, although we have plenty of food in Western countries, we are lacking in vitamins. Most people don't get enough vitamins because they choose foods that have been depleted of their nutritional essence. And those on low-calorie diets who are starving themselves do even worse. Organic vegetables, fruits, and fibre-rich foods retain their vitamin content, and yet very few people in Western countries consume those foods.

According to a 1992 study by Professor Cloarec, 37 percent of French people never eat fruit and 32 percent never eat green vegetables. In other Western countries, especially North America, the situation is similar. There's no doubt that a steady diet of fast-food, over-refined cereals and breads lacks essential vitamins. Since our bodies cannot manufacture most vitamins, food becomes the only source. And if we don't eat proper foods, our bodies suffer. There are two kinds of vitamins:

1. Water-soluble (or hydro soluble) vitamins that are used immediately, and are not stored within the body: vitamins B, C and PP.

2. Fat-soluble (or liposoluble) vitamins that can be stored in the body: vitamins A, D, E, and K.

VITAMIN DEFICIENCY

After the Second World War, Western societies experienced a boom in their populations. More people migrated to the cities, leaving fewer and fewer people to farm the lands. For the first time in history, food was not being eaten in the places where it was being grown. The population explosion required more food production.

Agricultural practices changed with the introduction of chemical fertilizers, pesticides, herbicides, and fungicides. In order to ship the food to the cities, conservation methods also changed. Additives and chemical preservatives became essential to food transport.

Eventually, over farming and chemicals depleted the soil, causing fruits and vegetables to gradually lose their nutritional value. Vitamins A, B1, B2, B3, and C have diminished by more than 30 percent in certain vegetables, depending on how they are grown. Vitamin E, for example, has practically disappeared from lettuce, peas, apples, and parsley, in much the same way that vitamin PP has vanished from strawberries. From one bunch of spinach to another (100g), the amount of vitamins can vary from 3 to 150 mg.

When white flour was introduced in the 19th century, people preferred it over coarse flours. That trend encouraged inventors to refine their techniques even more. In 1875, the discovery of the cylinder-run mill spelled the beginning of the end for whole-grain breads.

Industrial refining stripped grains of their essence: fibre, protein, essential fatty acids, vitamins, minerals, and trace elements. When white bread is kneaded by industrial beaters, the result is nothing more than pure starch with very little nutritional value.

Since the 1970s, there has been a return to organic farming, in which grains are germinated and planted in rich soils without pesticides and herbicides. Hopefully, this trend will grow and more and more people will opt for whole-grain organic breads over white.

OTHER MEANS OF VITAMIN DEPLETION

Once fruits and vegetables are harvested, they are subjected to many factors that deplete their vitamin content, especially vitamin C: exposure to air, storage, the length of time it takes to get the produce from the farm to the store and overcooking.

DIETING AND VITAMIN DEPLETION

Low-calorie diets are the worst offenders. When you restrict your food intake, you're also restricting the amount of vitamins you get.

LOW-CALORIE DIETS (1,500 A DAY)

Vitamins	Percentage of daily value obtained
A	30%
E	60%
B1	40%
B2	48%
B6	49%
C	45%
PP	43%
B5	40%
B9	38%

PRESERVING VITAMINS IN FOOD

Here are several suggestions on how to shop, store and cook your foods to retain as many vitamins as possible.

- Buy fresh produce on a daily basis
- Wash and soak your vegetables sparingly
- Eat raw vegetables and fruits
- Keep peels on when possible
- Avoid grating raw carrots, cabbage, etc.
- Cook foods quickly over low heat
- Steam or sauté vegetables
- Choose organic foods when possible
- Roast or grill meats, poultry, fish
- Buy frozen instead of canned foods
- Save vitamin-rich soup stock
- Keep milk out of light
- Avoid eating and reheating leftovers

SOURCES AND SIGNS OF VITAMIN DEPLETION

VITAMIN	Sources	Signs of deficiency
A (retinol)	Liver, egg yolks, milk, butter, carrots, spinach, tomatoes, apricots	Difficulty with night vision Sensitivity to light, dry skin Easily sunburned, ear, nose and throat infections
Provitamin A (betacarotene)	Carrots, watercress, spinach, mango, cantaloupe, apricots, broccoli, peaches, butter	Children: rickets Elderly: osteoporosis, bone demineralization
D (calciferol)	Liver, tuna, sardines, egg yolks, mushrooms, butter, cheese, the sun	Muscular fatigue, cardiovascular risk, skin aging
E (tocopherol)	Oils, hazelnuts, almonds, whole grains, milk, butter, eggs, dark chocolate, whole-wheat bread	Nose bleeds, hemorrhaging
K (menadione)	Made by bacteria in colon Liver, cabbage, spinach, eggs, broccoli, meat, cauliflower	Fatigue, irritability, memory loss, lack of appetite, depression, muscular weakness
B1 (thiamin)	Yeast, wheat germ, pork, giblets, fish, whole grains, whole-wheat bread	Seborrhoea, acne rosacea, light sensitivity, dull lifeless hair, lip and tongue sores
B2 (riboflavin)	Yeast, liver, kidneys, cheese, almonds, eggs, fish, milk, cocoa	Fatigue, insomnia, anorexia, depression, lesions of the skin and mucous membranes
PP (or B3, niacin, nicotinic acid)	Yeast, wheat bran, liver, meat, kidneys, fish, whole-wheat bread, dates, legumes, intestinal flora	
B5 (panthothenic acid)	Yeast, liver, kidneys, eggs, meat, mushrooms, grains, legumes	Fatigue, headache, nausea, vomiting, moodiness, low blood pressure, hair loss
B6 (pyridoxine)	Yeast, wheat germ, soy, liver, kidneys, meat, fish, brown rice, avocados, legumes, whole-wheat bread	Fatigue, depression, irritability, vertigo, nausea, skin lesions, sugar, cravings, headaches
B8 (biotin or vitamin H)	Intestinal flora, yeast, liver, kidneys, chocolate, aggs, mushrooms, chic-ken, cauliflower, legumes, meat, whole-wheat bread	Fatigue, loss of apetite, nausea, muscular weakness, oily skin, hair loss, insomnia, depression, neurological problems
B9 (folic acid)	Yeast, liver, oysters, soy, spinach, watercress, green vegetables, legu-mes, whole-wheat bread, cheese, milk, wheat germ	Fatigue, memory loss, insomnia, depression, mental confusion, slow healing, neurological problems
B12 (cyano-cobalamine)	Liver, kidneys, oysters, herring, fish, meat, eggs	Fatigue, irritability, palor, anaemia, loss of appetite, insomnia, neuromus-cular pain, memory loss, depression
C (ascorbic acid)	Rosehips, black currants, parsley, kiwi, broccoli, green vegetables, citrus fruits, liver, kidneys Fatigue, drowsiness, loss of appetite, muscular pain, multiple infections, shortness of breath	

MINERALS AND TRACE ELEMENTS

The body relies on a variety of chemical interactions in order to function properly. Mineral and trace elements are key to these interactions. Sodium and potassium are essential to nerve transmission. Calcium is important to the movement of muscles and iodine is the basis of thyroid hormones. Iron is necessary for the oxygenation of blood, and chromium helps the assimilation of glucose. When you lack minerals and trace elements, you can begin to suffer from physical problems. For example, a manganese deficiency encourages hypoglycemia. And a lack of nickel, chromium, and zinc contributes to insulin resistance.

Main categories of micronutrients:

- Minerals: calcium, phosphorus, potassium, sodium, sulfur, magnesium, etc.
- Trace elements: chromium, cobalt, zinc, copper, selenium, etc.

SHOULD YOU TAKE SUPPLEMENTS?

You'd think that the best way to get the minerals and trace elements that you need is through supplements. But you have to remember that supplements are artificially made. As such, they are not easily absorbed in the intestines. The best way to get all the minerals and trace elements you need is through healthy, whole foods. Fresh vegetables, fruits, legumes, and whole grains are the best sources. The only supplements I recommend are brewer's yeast and wheat germ, which contain the minerals and trace elements needed to lower glycemia and insulinemia, which in turn help you to lose weight. At breakfast on alternating days, add 15 ml (1 tsp.) of brewer's yeast or wheat germ to a dairy product like yogurt.

RECOMMENDED SUPPLEMENTS

For 100 g (3.5 oz.)	Brewer's yeast	Wheat germ
Water	6 g	11 g
Proteins	42 g	26 g
Carbohydrates	19 g	34 g
Lipids	2 g	10 g
Fibre	22 g	17 g
Potassium	1,800 mg	850 mg
Magnesium	230 mg	260 mg
Phosphorus	1,700 mg	1,100 mg
Calcium	100 mg	70 mg
Iron	18 mg	9 mg
Beta Carotene	0.01 mg	0 mg
Vitamin B1	10 mg	2 mg
Vitamin B2	5 mg	0.7 mg
Vitamin B5	12 mg	1.7 mg
Vitamin B6	4 mg	3 mg
Vitamin B12	0.01 mg	0 mg
Folic acid	4 mg	430 mg
Vitamin PP	46 mg	4.5 mg
Vitamin E	0 mg	21 mg

CHAPTER 8:
DANGEROUS SIDE EFFECTS OF POOR EATING HABITS: HIGH CHOLESTEROL AND HEART DISEASE

Heart disease is the N°1 killer of both men and women in Western societies, despite extensive educational campaigns to prevent it. Nevertheless, most of us are familiar with the risk factors: high cholesterol, high blood pressure, diabetes, obesity, smoking, lack of exercise and stress. A family history of heart disease also increases your risk. On the Montignac Method, the goal is to lose weight in a healthy manner. Not only do you eat low-GI carbohydrates, but you are also advised to watch the kinds of fats you consume.

CHOLESTEROL: A MALIGNED SUBSTANCE

Cholesterol is a naturally occurring, waxy substance essential to the smooth functioning of our bodies. It helps the body produce hormones and digests fats. Up to 75 percent of cholesterol is actually made by the body; the remaining 25 percent is derived from food, specifically the fats you consume: saturated, mono or polyunsaturated foods.

THE GOOD AND THE BAD

Cholesterol does not float around freely in your bloodstream. Instead, it attaches itself to two kinds of proteins: low density lipoproteins (LDLs) or high density lipoproteins (HDL).

LDLs distribute cholesterol to cells, especially the cells of artery walls, where fatty deposits form. LDL cholesterol has been characterized as the "bad cholesterol" because over time the cholesterol on artery walls turns into plaque that blocks the flow of blood. This artery obstruction can cause cardiovascular problems such as angina, heart attack, and stroke.

HDL cholesterol, on the other hand, is known as the good cholesterol, because it actually scrubs out the cholesterol plaque on artery walls. The higher the levels of HDL the less risk of cardiovascular problems there is.

CHOLESTEROL LEVELS

Heart specialists have created much more stringent guidelines for cholesterol levels than a few decades ago.

When you go for a check-up, your doctor will look at three cholesterol measurements:

- Total cholesterol (HDL + LDL): must be less than or equal to 2 grams per liter of blood

- LDL cholesterol: must be less than 130 grams per liter of blood

- HDL cholesterol: must be greater than 0.45 grams per liter of blood for men and 0.55 grams per liter for women

CARDIOVASCULAR RISKS

Cardiovascular risk is doubled if your total cholesterol level reaches 2.2 grams per liter of blood, and by four times if it is greater than 2.60 grams per liter. Yet it has been observed that 15 percent of heart attacks occurred in patients whose percentage of total cholesterol was less than two grams per liter. So it seems that the overall recommended cholesterol levels are not what is significant, but rather the ratio of LDL to HDL cholesterol.

Cholesterol is only one risk factor in heart disease. Here are the others: hyperglycemia (with or without diabetes), hyperinsulinism, hypertriglyceridemia, antioxidant deficiency (vitamins A, C and E, beta-carotene, zinc, copper, selenium, and polyphenols), and smoking. In many cases, diet and lifestyle can correct these problems.

CHANGE YOUR DIET

High cholesterol can be treated by modern drugs, but there are other things you can do to help. Here are some suggestions:

1. Lose excess weight: Weight loss leads to improved health on many levels. Cholesterol levels usually improve, especially if you limit your intake of saturated fats in such food as fatty meat and butter. It is saturated fats that raise your cholesterol levels.

2. Watch cholesterol-laden food: Egg yolks, giblets, and coconut oil contain critical levels of cholesterol. The World Health Organization has been advising for a long time that total recommended cholesterol intake should be restricted to 300 mg a day. However, recent studies have refuted that advice. A daily intake of 1,000 mg of cholesterol only leads to about a five percent rise in cholesterol. So you can relax a bit about the cholesterol content of food. On the other hand, you must keep in mind the amount of saturated fats you consume—they are the ones that raise your cholesterol.

AMOUNT OF SATURATED FATS

	Lipids for 100 g	Saturated fats
Lean cooked ham*	3 g	1.1 g
Smoked ham*	13 g	1.7 g
Head cheese*	13 g	4.6 g
Foie gras**	45 g	17 g
Dry sausage**	30 g	12.1 g
Bacon**	31 g	11.1 g
Blood pudding**	34 g	12.6 g
Mortadella cheese	30 g	12.4 g
Pork liver pâté**	37 g	15 g
Salami**	42 g	16.4 g
Frankfurters**	24 g	10 g

* Meats with little fat.

**Very fatty meats. To be avoided or only very moderately consumed.

3. Choose your fats carefully

There are several kinds of fats:

• **Saturated fats**. These are found especially in meats, very fatty pork products, whole dairy products, cheese, and palm oil. These fats raise your total cholesterol level, especially LDL cholesterol. Chicken, with its skin removed, has little effect on cholesterol levels.

• **Polyunsaturated fish oils.** It is a well-known fact that Arctic peoples like the Inuit, who eat a lot of fatty fish, enjoy a life free of cardiovascular problems. We now know that fish oils are the main reason. Fish oils like omega-3 significantly lower triglycerides, a risk factor in heart disease. Salmon, sardines, mackerel, anchovies, and herring all contain heart-healthy oils.

• **Polyunsaturated vegetable oils**. Sunflower, corn, soy, peanut, soy, and rapeseed oils all contain linoleic acid. Polyunsaturated fatty acids are also found in walnuts, almonds, peanuts, and sesame seeds. The problem with polyunsaturated fatty acids is that they oxidize very easily. Oxidation especially occurs when the body lacks antioxidants (see chart on page X). Thus, polyunsaturated vegetable fats can be as bad for your heart as saturated fatty acids if you don't consume a diet that includes a full complement of antioxidants.

• **Unsaturated transfatty acids.** These are fatty acids that are by-products of food processing of mono- or polyunsaturated fatty acids: margarine, industrial bread, cookies, pastries, candy, and instant meals. Transfatty acids are just as dangerous as saturated fats. It's better, then, to eat home-cooked meals than to rely on over processed foods.

• **Monounsaturated fatty acids.** A prime example of a monounsaturated fatty acid is oleic acid, which is found in poultry (goose and duck fat) and foie gras, but especially in olive oil. Olive oil is the champion of fats because it has a positive effect on cholesterol: it lowers LDL and raises HDL.

4. Choose your carbohydrates wisely

Hypoglycemia and hyperinsulinism are major risks to heart health. Choosing carbohydrates with a high GI, such as potatoes, white flour and sugar, can spell trouble for your heart. Rather, choose low-GI carbohydrates such as lentils, peas, chickpeas, fruit, green vegetables, and whole-grain cereals. If you have high triglycerides, you should also watch your intake of high-GI carbohydrates and alcohol.

5. Eat more fibre

Fibre in such foods as oats and legumes aids in the effective digestion and metabolism of fats. Pectin, in apples, for example, also leads to a slight drop in cholesterol levels.

6. Fill up on antioxidants

Oxidation of foods leads to the release of free radicals. Free radicals alter cells and have been linked to the aging process and cancer. Free radicals can be controlled by eating foods rich in antioxidants: vitamin A and beta-carotene, vitamin C, vitamin E, selenium, zinc, copper and polyphenols, which are found in red wine. (See antioxidant chart below.)

FOODS RICH IN ANTIOXIDANTS

Vitamin E	Vitamin C	Beta-carotene	Copper
wheat germ oil	rosehips	raw carrots	oysters
corn oil	black currants	watercress	beef liver
soya oil	parsley	spinach	veal liver
sunflower oil	kiwi	mango	mutton liver
peanut oil	broccoli	cantaloupe	mussels
rapeseed oil	sorrel	apricots	cocoa powder
olive oil	raw green/red peppers	broccoli	wheat germ
wheat germ	tarragon	peaches	white beans
hazelnuts, almonds	raw white/red cabbage	tomatoes	hazelnuts
germinated grains	watercress	oranges	dried peas
walnuts, peanuts	lemon, orange	dandelion	oatmeal
wild rice		parsley	walnuts sweetbreads
Vitamin A	**Selenium**	**Zinc**	**Polyphenols**
codliver oil	oysters	oysters	wine
liver	chicken liver	dried peas	grape seeds
butter	beef liver	duck liver	green tea
cooked eggs	fish	brewer's yeast	olive oil
fresh apricots	eggs	legumes	onions
cheese	mushrooms	kidneys	apples
salmon	onions	eel	
whole milk	whole-wheat bread	lentils	
sardines	brown rice	meat	
sour cream	lentils sweetbreads	whole-wheat bread	

7. Drink wine

Studies by Professors Masquelier and Renaud have shown that consuming one to three glasses of wine (especially red) per day reduces cardiovascular risk. In effect, wine contains substances that lower LDL cholesterol (bad cholesterol) and raise HDL cholesterol (good cholesterol). It protects the artery walls and makes the blood flow more easily, preventing thrombosis.

8. Improve your lifestyle

Stress, smoking, and lack of exercise also have a negative effect on cholesterol. Take time to relax by listening to music, enjoying your favourite hobby, learning meditation, or practising yoga. Smoking constricts your blood vessels, and if they are clogged by cholesterol, you increase your risk of cardiovascular disease. And by all means, try to start a regular exercise program to strengthen your heart. Do what you love to do. Is it golfing? Tennis? Riding a bike? It will keep you motivated. Speak to your doctor before you start.

TIPS TO IMPROVE YOUR HEART HEALTH

- Lose weight if you are overweight or obese
- Choose fish and poultry (without skin) more often
- Restrict your meat consumption (max. 5 oz/140g. per day)
- Choose lean meats only

- Eat only small amounts of butter and margarine (max. 15 ml or 1 tbsp. daily)
- Reduce your cheese consumption
- Drink skim milk and eat fat-free dairy products
- Avoid high GI carbohydrates such as potatoes, white flour and sugar
- Increase your consumption of low GI, high-fibre carbohydrates such as fruit, whole grains, vegetables and legumes
- Increase your consumption of mono- and polyunsaturated vegetable oils (olive, sunflower and rapeseed)
- Boost your antioxidant and chromium intake
- Drink red wine (optional)
- Control stress
- Exercise regularly
- Stop smoking

CHAPTER 9:
SUGAR IS POISON

I believe that sugar has harmed humans as much as excessive use of alcohol and tobacco combined. International medical conferences of diabetes experts, psychiatrists and dentists, among others, have warned of the dangers of sugar. Sugar was practically non-existent in ancient times. The Greeks did not even have a word for it. Around 325 BC, Alexander the Great, who had conquered the lands at the plains of the Indus, described sugar as "a sort of honey found in canes and reeds growing at the water's edge." The Roman Emperor Nero was the first to know saccharum.

But by the 7th century AD, sugar cane was cultivated in Persia and Sicily. Gradually, Arabs began to acquire a taste for it. In 1653, a German scholar, Dr. Rauwolf, noted the change in the Arab population: "The Turks and the Moors are no longer the intrepid soldiers they had been before they discovered sugar.» The Crusades introduced sugar to the Europeans. The Spanish began to cultivate it in the southern reaches of their country soon after. The New World brought new reserves and the sugar trade began in earnest. Portugal, Spain, and England became rich by trading sugar for slaves. They, in turn, planted, grew, and harvested the plentiful fields of sugar cane in the southern United States. France, too, built a number of sugar refineries by the 1700s.

Napoleon was instrumental in finding the technique of extracting sugar from beets. The defeat of Napoleon at the Battle of Trafalgar in 1805 and the continental blockade that resulted led him to encourage the production of sugar from beets. By 1812, the discovery of the extraction procedure by Benjamin Delessert made it possible to do so. Just 25 years later, France enjoyed a surplus of sugar, but its consumption had still not reached the levels it is at today.

By 1880, the French were consuming the equivalent of five sugar cubes a day, 17 pounds (8kg) a year. At the turn of the century, it had more than doubled to 37 pounds (17kg) per year. Today it has reached almost 83 pounds (38kg) per person per year. Still the Europeans are far from being the worst offenders. North Americans, especially Americans, eat an astonishing 130 pounds (59kg) of sugar per person per year—and growing.

Sugar is often hidden in the many foods that we eat. It's unnecessarily added to canned vegetables, potato chips, soups, sauces and the like. In 1970 the amount of sugar indirectly absorbed (through beverages, sweets, preserves, etc.) was 58 percent of total sugar consumption. By 1980 it had risen to more than 65 percent. A two-litre bottle of cola contains the equivalent of about 46 sugar cubes.

North Americans often have soft drinks with their meals. That's because of the influence of powerful advertising campaigns by major soft-drink manufacturers. Developing countries are also targeted. In these countries, the population's basic nutritional needs are not even being met, and yet they are consuming litres of nutritionless, sweet beverages every year. Sugar-filled ice cream and other frozen desserts used to be served only at special occasions.

Now they are eaten on a frequent basis through vending machines and fast-food outlets. Junk food is also easily accessible from vending machines in public places and supermarkets. It takes a hero to avoid the temptation at every corner. We all know that sugar causes a host of health problems. Excessive sugar consumption (like eating a lot of high GI carbohydrates) can cause an increase in cardiovascular risk, due to hyperglycemia, hyperinsulinism, and hypertriglyceridemia[16].

Dr. Yudkin points to the East African tribes Mascar and Samburee, whose high-fat diets are almost completely devoid of

---

[16] Epidemiological studies conducted over 12 years by Professor W. Willett of Harvard's School of Public Health have clearly shown the link between sugar and the prevalence of obesity and diabetes in the United States. And, according to Dr. Edward Ciovannucci, also of Harvard University, 23 epidemiological studies show a correlation between excessive sugar consumption and colon cancer.

sugar. As a result, cardiovascular disease is almost nonexistent. On the other hand, the residents of St. Helena Island, who eat lots of sugar and very little fat, suffer from a great many coronary diseases.

Dental cavities due to excessive sugar consumption are so widespread in Western countries that the World Health Organization ranks dental and oral diseases third among the top health problems afflicting Western society today. (Heart disease and cancer are first and second, respectively.) Excess sugar consumption is often linked to diabetes. But it is not true that diabetes only affects those with a family history. Not all adult diabetics are obese, but most are.

Unfortunately, the United States has one of the highest rates of obesity in the world, a direct consequence of a diet rich in bad carbohydrates, especially sugar. Having read the previous chapters, you now understand that sugar, a purely chemical product, can cause hypoglycemia, generally upset metabolism and provoke a number of digestive disorders.

Vitamin B1 deficiency can be caused by excess sugar consumption. Large quantities of this vitamin are needed to absorb carbohydrates. Sugar, just like all refined starches (white flour, white rice, etc.), is completely devoid of vitamin B1, creating a deficit whose consequences generally include nervous exhaustion, fatigue, depression, muscle fatigue and loss of concentration, memory and perception. This may also be the root of children's difficulties in school.

ARTIFICIAL SWEETENERS

I strongly suggest that you wean yourself from sugar as much as possible. Of course, it will be hidden in foods, but if you are able to cut back or totally eliminate granulated sugar and sugar cubes from your diet, you will be successful. You have two options: the right one: give it up or the wrong one: replace it with artificial sweeteners. There are four major artificial sweeteners. None of them, except polyols, have any nutritional value.

1. Saccharine: Discovered in 1879, this is the oldest sugar substitute. It is not used by the body and has a sweetening potential of more than 350 times that of the saccharose in natural sugar. It has the advantage of being very stable in acidic substances and can tolerate medium temperatures. Canada, however, has banned it. Saccharine was the most commercialized sweetener until the discovery of aspartame.

2. Cyclamates: Even though their discovery dates back to 1937, cyclamates are not nearly as well known as saccharine. They are less sweet than saccharine and they leave an aftertaste. Cyclamates, however, resist high temperatures. The most commonly used cyclamate is made from sodium cyclamate. Other kinds include calcium cyclamate and cyclamate acid.

3. Aspartame: In Chicago in 1965, James Schlatter, a researcher at Searle Laboratories, discovered aspartame. This sugar substitute is a combination of two natural amino acids: aspartic acid and phenylalanine. Its sweetening potential is 180 to 200

times that of saccharose. It has no bitter aftertaste, and several taste tests have attested to its natural flavour. More than 60
countries use it in the production of food and drink products.
Artificial sweeteners have stirred controversy ever since their
introduction. Saccharine, for one, has been suspected of causing cancer. Cyclamates have also been linked to cancer and
were outlawed in the United States in 1969. As for aspartame,
it has been the subject of numerous controversies since its discovery. Still, many studies have proven that it is free of toxins,
even when consumed in high doses. The U.S. Food and Drug
Administration has officially recognized this fact. Aspartame is
available in two forms: in tablets that rapidly dissolve in hot or
cold beverages and in powder form, particularly recommended
for desserts and other recipes.

One tablet of aspartame is as sweet as a 0.2-ounce (6g) sugar
cube and contains 0.004 ounces (11mg) of absorbable carbohydrates. In powder form, one teaspoon is as sweet as one teaspoon of sugar and contains 0.14 ounces (4g) of absorbable carbohydrates. The World Health Organization has set the accepted
daily amount at one tablet per pound of body weight. In other
words, a person weighing 120 pounds (54kg) could consume
up to 120 tablets in one day without noting any toxic, long-term
effects.

Even though artificial sweeteners are said non-toxic, they could
seriously disturb metabolism in the long run. Here's how: When
the body perceives a sweet taste, it prepares itself to digest carbohydrates, then cannot find them. If sweeteners are used during

the day, any intake of real carbohydrates during those 24 hours could lead to abnormal hyperglycemia, followed by hypoglycemia. After the body has been frustrated by artificial sweeteners, it could compensate for this situation by excessively absorbing carbohydrates in the intestines.

This increased digestion of carbohydrates leads to hyperglycemia (greater than that which normally occurs for the carbohydrate in question), which, by way of the hyperinsulinism set off by it, then leads to hypoglycemia. As hyperinsulinism is a factor in the storage of fats, and hypoglycemia causing a premature return to the sensation of hunger, we should ask if using artificial sweeteners does not indirectly cause weight gain. Besides, the widespread use of aspartame over the last 30 years certainly hasn't kept obesity under control, now has it?

The craving for sugar seems universal, then. If it isn't innate, then it must be acquired while we are still in the womb. And then, as we grow up, we are bombarded by foods chock-full of sugar. All of this is aided and abetted by parents who want to show their love and reward their children with sweets. I suggest parents discourage children from developing a love of sugar. Teach them instead to enjoy sour and bitter tastes as well. To wean them from their sugar cravings, you can use artificially flavoured sodas as a substitute to help them make the transition from sugary sodas to water for children and adolescents who are "addicted" to sugar. Water is actually the only beverage a child should drink with lunch and dinner. At snack time, fruit juice and/or water are clearly better than soda.

4. Polyols: Polyols are another kind of artificial sweetener (also known as sorbitol, mannitol, xylose, maltose, lactilol, lycasin, or polydextrose). They appear in products such as chocolate, chewing gum, and candy. Unfortunately, the only advantage polyols have, compared to sugar is that they do not cause cavities. They do, however, release fatty acids that are reabsorbed by the colon. They can even promote, because of fermentation in the colon, bloating, and diarrhea. However, their GI varies anywhere from 20 to 65. The GI of mannitol for instance is one of the lowest.

5. Fructose: Fructose is not an artificial sweetener because it has been classified as a "natural sugar." It also has a low GI (20), which helps the weight-loss cause. Finally, it has almost the same density as the saccharose in sugar, which makes it handy for baking. However, one must be very careful to choose the real fructose made from beet or sugar cane because most of the products sold by supermarkets are a fake fructose which is in fact a chemical product (oligo-glucose) made from corn starch and whose GI range from 60 to 70 according to its concentration. Nevertheless, obese people and diabetics must use very moderate amounts because it has been shown that large quantities can raise triglyceride levels.

CHAPTER 10:
KEEPING CHILDREN HEALTHY WITH GOOD FOODS

From infancy to young adulthood, children require a proper diet of whole grains, fruits, vegetables and proteins. How they eat in childhood will determine how they eat for the rest of their lives. Illness and food allergies can often throw off a child's appetite. If these conditions are not addressed quickly, then poor eating habits may result. But certain illnesses can be caused or aggravated by the foods children eat. In this case, their diets should be re-evaluated. Even though there is an abundance of food in Western industrialized societies, the quality is deteriorating rapidly.

THE DEMISE OF QUALITY FOODS

Convenience is at the root of today's lack of quality food. Due to our frantic pace, we often just open a can of noodles or a box of crackers to feed our children. We want all of the advantages of our modern society without the inconvenience: We want to have our cake and eat it too. Of course, I recognize that there are times when it is necessary to get our children out the door to their soccer or ballet lessons. But what I'm against is the daily use of convenience foods. Remember, processed food is nutritionally inferior to fresh, homemade meals. Good health in children can only be supported through sound nutrition.

FOODS TO WATCH

Bread
White bread should be eliminated from children's diets. Refined flour is devoid of minerals, especially magnesium and vitamin B1, which is indispensable to the digestion of carbohydrates. B1 deficiency can also cause fatigue. Whole-wheat and whole-grain bread contain vitamins, minerals, and trace elements that children require for good nutrition.

Starches
Children whose bodies are of average weight and height normally tolerate carbohydrates well. Starches, therefore, can provide a good source of nutrition for them. But that does not mean you should heap on high-GI carbohydrates such as potatoes and corn. If you have difficulty thinking up new menus without French fries, turn back to Chapter 4 for ideas. There are plenty of new vegetables to choose from. By offering your children variety, they'll begin to develop new tastes and seek out new foods.

Pasta is one of children's favourite foods. While wholegrain pastas are preferable, you can also serve spaghetti and tagliatelle, cooked *al dente*. These are both low-GI carbohydrates. Avoid ravioli, macaroni, and other pastas made from "soft" wheat; they are high-GI carbohydrates. Again brown rice is preferable, but Basmati rice will also do. Serve these rices with vegetables such as tomatoes, zucchini, eggplant, among others, like they do in India. Lentils are also a good accompaniment to rice.

Fruit
Children are able to eat fruit after meals without any digestive problems. However, if you notice your child suffering from stomach aches, bloating, or gas, you may want to save fruit for snack time or first thing in the morning instead.

Beverages
Water is by far the best liquid for children. Sweet beverages such as soft drinks and concentrated juices should be avoided. (Freshly squeezed juices with the pulp are okay because they retain their vitamins, minerals, and fibre.) I believe that sugared drinks are poisonous for children; it's the equivalent to excess alcohol consumption in adults. Exceptions can be made for special occasions, but don't make them a habit. Colas are the worst offenders. They contain phosphoric acid, loads of sugar and caffeine. Sugar can also be found in syrups and powdered drink mixes. When children become used to the taste of sugar, they crave it. Milk at meals is not fine and should be served at breakfast only because of its insulinotropic effect.

Sugar and sweets

I don't recommend banning sugar from your children's diets altogether, but I do suggest you restrict it as much as possible. But be aware that sugar crops up in so many children's foods, from breakfast cereals to cookies and ice cream. Avoid, without forbidding, sweets, candy, and chocolate bars, which comprise as much as 80 percent sugar. Reread Chapter 9 to firm your resolve.

Above all, don't let sugar rule your home. Explain to your children why sugar is not good for them. Whatever you do, don't feed water sugar to your newborn infants, a common practice in hospitals. When candies and sweets are given to your children as gifts, don't make a fuss over it, but try to discreetly get rid of them as soon as possible. Remember, too, that vitamin B1 deficiency, which sugar causes, interferes with proper digestion of carbohydrates, resulting in fatigue, difficulty concentrating, attention and memory lapses, and even some forms of depression in children. Your child's school work will naturally suffer.

CHILDREN AND ARTIFICIAL SWEETENERS

If your child is truly overweight, I recommend you Stevia, agave syrup or fructose, say on a yogurt or in hot cocoa, because they are natural products and have no effects on glycemia.

MEALS

Here are suggestions to bring quality into your children's meals:

• Avoid high-GI carbohydrates. As explained previously, they cause the body to secrete abnormal amounts of insulin. Hyperinsulinism can lead to weight gain, diabetes, and heart disease.
• Serve balanced meals over the entire day. Include proteins, carbohydrates, and lipids.

Breakfast

Breakfast is the most important meal of the day, especially for children. A breakfast full of low-GI carbohydrates is your best bet:

• Whole-wheat bread with a little butter or sugar-free peanut butter
• Multi-grain, sugar-free cereal. Avoid cornflakes and any other cereal containing corn, rice, sugar, honey or caramel coating
• Fresh fruit
• Sugar-free preserves
• Dairy products (milk, plain yogurt with fresh fruit)
• Honey and maple syrup should be used sparingly because it is a high-GI carbohydrate

Lunch

Proteins should be served at noon: meat, poultry, or fish. Avoid serving high-GI carbohydrates with these proteins, especially French fries, baked or mashed potatoes. However, potatoes boiled in their skins and sweet potatoes are acceptable.

Vegetables such as beans, lentils, peas, and chickpeas can also be served, along with small amounts of Basmati rice or semolina. Cooked carrots are acceptable for children. Side dishes should include fibre-rich vegetables such as green beans, cauliflower, mushrooms, tomatoes, etc.

Vary the menu so that children don't fall into the same routine meals every day. Pack them healthy lunches. If they eat cafeteria food, try to find out what the menus are in advance. If your child is of average weight, though, you don't need to worry unnecessarily. Just make the proper adjustments at dinner.

Snacks

Frequent meals are preferable for children because they require so much energy in their daily lives. That's why snacks are perfectly acceptable. Fruits make excellent snacks, as does whole-wheat bread with a little butter or sugar-free peanut butter. Quality chocolate bars made with 70 percent cocoa are also acceptable.

Dinner

Like lunch, dinner should include meat, fish, eggs, or even "good" carbohydrates such as lentils, Basmati rice, or pasta. Start out the meal with a chunky soup of leeks, tomatoes, celery, broccoli, cauliflower, etc. Soups are an excellent way to get your children to eat vegetables, which are essential to proper digestion and bowel function. They also contain essential vitamins, minerals, and fibre. Stuffing vegetables is also another way to get your kids to eat them. Stuff green peppers, tomatoes, eggplant, artichokes, or cabbage with brown rice or whole-wheat bread crumbs. They'll love it.

Low-fat dairy products, such as custard, pudding, and crème caramel, can be served for dessert. Plain yogurt with a little sugar-free jam or preserves also makes an acceptable dessert. Occasionally, you can serve a piece of cake. Hotdogs and hamburgers should be banned from your home. They contain high-GI carbohydrates and loads of saturated fats, both of which are very unhealthy for your children.

Occasionally, you can use fast-food hamburgers and hotdogs for quick meals, but please do not make a habit out of them. Better yet, reward your children with a grand meal out at a fancy French restaurant! Fast food at home doesn't always have to mean bad food. In fact, you can make your own whole-wheat pizzas with fresh vegetables. Whole-wheat pita or tortilla wraps can be filled with red peppers, lettuce, tomatoes, and beans. A spaghetti meal with tomato sauce is nutritious and fast. And a whole-wheat sandwich of ham, cheese, or fish with a little to-mato and lettuce is also a good choice.

SPECIAL CASES OVERWEIGHT CHILDREN

A few extra pounds on your son or daughter do not make them obese. Try to remain calm about your child's excess weight. Never attempt to put your child on a low-calorie diet because it can be dangerous to his or her health. Your doctor will assure you that most children lose those extra pounds once they reach adolescence. But be aware that excess weight in children is an indicator that something may be wrong with their metabolism.

The excess weight may signal poor glucose tolerance. If it is ad-dressed in time, you may be able to help your child re-establish an average weight. In this case, the Montignac Method can be applied (see Chapter 4). Choose low-GI carbohydrates. If your child should eat a high-GI carbohydrate, quickly compensate by serving a low-GI carbohydrate to keep the glycemia in check.

Overweight children should also be encouraged to exercise because it has been proven to reduce or eliminate weight pro-blems. Kids who are typically overweight tend to spend a lot of time in front of the TV or computers. Not only aren't they get-ting adequate exercise, but watching TV encourages snacking on unhealthy treats. Overweight boys grow into overweight tee-nagers. Girls can start out slim but gain weight at puberty due to their hormones. Fluctuations in hormones during puberty, pregnancy, and menopause can cause changes in metabolism. Many adolescent females and women constantly worry about their weight. Often, they subject themselves to crash diets. They essentially starve themselves, many of them reaching the stage of anorexia, bulimia, or depression. A healthy alternative is to use the Montignac Method. By doing so, they can adopt healthy but slimming eating habits, and regain their vitality and sense of power to help them feel confident in the world.

TIRED CHILDREN

It is shocking when you hear children and adolescents complain about how tired they are. I blame their high-GI carbohydrate diets. When they eat sugary cereals in the morning, by 11:00 they'll already feel lethargic. They may have difficulty concentrating, may yawn excessively, and not be able to do their work. And it doesn't stop there. By mid-afternoon, after a lunch of hotdogs, French fries and a sugary soft-drink, they'll slump over their desks in fatigue. Late-afternoon snacks of sweets and cookies further deplete their energy levels. Why not serve them fresh fruits, whole grains, and vegetables instead? Watch how they'll perk up. You'll be glad you did.

CHAPTER 11:
EXERCISE

On any given day on the streets of North America, you'll see hordes of people jogging at daybreak, at noon or after work. This is great for cardiovascular health, but it won't necessarily keep these enthusiasts from turning into the Michelin Man if their diets don't include nutritious, low-fat, high-fibre foods.

Exercise doesn't have to be strenuous to do good. Parisians, for example, make it a habit of strolling through the Bois de Boulogne or the Jardins des Tuileries for their exercise. However, even the French are not immune to the new thinking. In 1999, a weekly French newspaper took a poll that showed 71 percent believed that exercise was the best way to lose weight. Once you see how much exercise it takes to work off two pounds of fat, you might change your mind.

EXERCISE TIME REQUIRED TO LOSE 2 LB. OF FAT

Steady exercise	Men (hours)	Women (hours)
Walking at a normal pace	138	246
Walking rapidly	63	96
Golf	36	47
Bicycling	30	38
Swimming (crawl)	17	21
Jogging	14	18
Tennis	13	16
Squash	8	11

Source: Dr. Mondenard

French research by Dr. Mondenard shows that in order to lose two pounds (1kg), a person would need to exercise for hours. A jogger wanting to lose 11 pounds (5kg), for example, would have to run for an hour and a half non-stop, five times a week.

ENDURANCE PAYS OFF

The only way to lose weight and keep it off is to exercise for prolonged periods of time at a steady pace. One hour of continuous exercise is much more effective than 30 minutes three times a day. At rest, the body uses fatty acids in the blood as well as adenosine triphosphate (ATP) in muscles for fuel. When you begin intense exercise, your body draws on the glycogen from your muscles for fuel. After 20 minutes, the body uses a combination of the glycogen and stored fats for energy. After 40 minutes, mostly fats are used in order to protect the remaining glycogen. That's when you start to burn up stored fat. The Montignac Method can also be adopted for those who exercise in order to avoid hypoglycemia. (Full-time athletes' requirements are more complex and cannot be addressed in this book.) With all exercise programs, you should consult your doctor before beginning. In all cases, start out slowly and build up your endurance.

EXERCISE IS HEALTHY FOR YOU

If you don't use it, you'll lose it. Exercise is important to your body's smooth functioning. Taken on gradually and with proper training, exercise can boost your health and mental outlook. It helps postpone aging by strengthening your cardiovascular system and can help to keep the weight off once you have lost it. Muscle gradually replaces fat, which helps you to feel stronger and healthier. Pretty soon you won't be the one to wait for the elevator; instead you'll take the stairs. You won't be the one to drive five minutes to the convenience store; you'll walk.

Exercise can also improve glucose tolerance and hyperinsulinism, which can cause hypoglycemia and obesity. Cholesterol and high blood pressure also improve with regular exercise. Mentally, your outlook will brighten and you'll regain a sense of youthfulness. A sense of well-being will return, too. Your metabolism will improve, which will help you to lose and maintain your weight.

KEEP A PERSPECTIVE

Exercise can become extreme, and in some cases, addictive. Don't overdo it. Drink plenty of water when exercising to keep you well-hydrated. By combining a healthy diet and reasonable physical exercise, you'll reach a level of peace and optimism.

CHAPTER 12:
CALCULATING YOUR IDEAL WEIGHT

When we step on a scale, what exactly are we weighing? Our total weight is comprised of our bones, muscles, fat, organs, viscera, nerves, and water. Fat makes up about 15 percent of men's weight, and about 22 percent of women's. Obesity occurs when we surpass our ideal weight by 20 percent. Still, it is very difficult to measure fat. Indeed, measuring instruments like calipers are far from accurate.

One way to get a clearer picture is to use the Lorentz method using centimetres and kilograms.

$$\text{Weight (men)} = (\text{Height} - 100) - \frac{(\text{Height} - 150)}{4}$$
$$\text{Weight (women)} = (\text{Height} - 100) - \frac{(\text{Height} - 140)}{2}$$

The Lorentz calculation, however, doesn't take into account age or skeletal structure, and it is not valid for women who measure less than 1.5 m (5 ft.). It is best to resort to the weight at which you feel best, which everyone senses intuitively.

The Quetelet index or body mass index (BMI) is more popular. It calculates the relationship between weight and height squared.

$$\text{Index} = \frac{\text{Weight (in kg)}}{\text{Height}^2 \text{ (in m}^2)}$$

The average BMI for men is between 20 and 25; for women, between 19 and 24. Overweight falls between 25 and 29. Thirty and up is considered obese. After 40, one is considered seriously obese and may have a serious medical problem. New weight scales on the market today measures weight and body fat. They are useful in helping you to monitor your fat loss. Ideally, you will want to lose body fat, not muscle. Body fat is deleterious to health depending upon where it appears on the body: above or below the navel. To measure this distribution, use this formula:

$$\frac{\text{Waist measurement (at the navel)}}{\text{Hip measurement (at the hips or fullest part)}}$$

CALCULATE YOUR BMI USING THE INDEX BELOW:

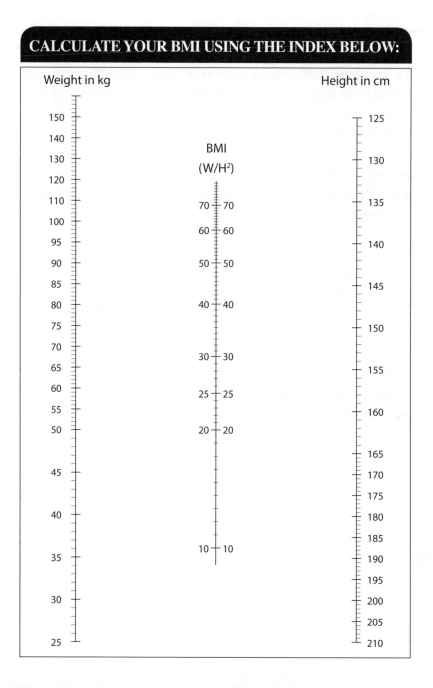

Weight in kg

BMI
(W/H²)

Height in cm

To find your BMI, place a ruler from your weight over to your height, and where the ruler hits the BMI is your number. Generally, the index is 0.85-1 for men and 0.65-0.85 for women. In androgenic obesity (also known as the apple shaped body), fat is concentrated above the navel, in the face, neck, chest and abdomen. The ratio is always greater than one. Diabetes, hypercholesterolemia, high blood pressure, and cardiovascular diseases are usually associated with this body shape.

In gynecoid obesity (also known as the pear-shaped body), most of the fatty mass is found below the navel in the lower body: hips, buttocks, thighs, and lower belly. The female body is typical of this shape. The risk of illness is less. As for your goal, look beyond the stringent insurance company measurements to find your ideal weight. Base it on what makes you feel comfortable and what you can achieve realistically and healthfully. Try to avoid making your objective out of reach because it will only serve to discourage you. If you're having trouble determining a healthy number for you, consult your doctor.

CONCLUSION

Archaeologists have now determined that the human species has been around for about four million years. Primitive peoples were primarily hunter/gatherers and their diet consisted of meats with lots of fat and high-fibre carbohydrates such as fruit in the summer and root vegetables during the fall and winter. It was essentially composed of low-GI carbohydrates.

In the Mesolithic period (10,000 BC), humans began to plant wild grains, which kicked off the agricultural era. Wheat and lentils were cultivated in Egypt, whereas oats, millet, rye, and buckwheat were grown in northern cimes by the Saxons and the Celts. Of course, these grains and legumes were consumed naturally with all their fibre intact. For centuries afterwards, those foods were the basis of the human diet.

From the 19th century on, however, the human diet changed forever. Flour was refined and sugar was introduced. Those two elements alone negatively impacted humans' digestive systems and metabolism. But because they were slowly integrated into the foods people ate, the deleterious effects were subtle.

In effect, it has been a slow poisoning, just as in the novel of François Mauriac, the case of Madame Thérèse Desqueyroud, who surreptitiously killed her husband by putting small doses of cyanide in his food over a long period of time.

By 1930, obesity had reached such a level in the United States that it finally caught the attention of medical researchers at such places as Michigan University. They, in turn, devised their calorie theory, and we've been off on the wrong track ever since.

Indeed, we have been starving ourselves with low-calorie diets and slowly poisoning our bodies with bad food for decades now. The consequence is a rise in obesity, diabetes, and hyperinsulinism.

It was during the Second World War that American troops were supplied with dehydrated potato flakes and preserved meats. Food had never undergone such processing before, which changed the way food has been prepared ever since.

These refined, over processed foods were made available after the war at army surplus stores, and it fuelled a trend that we've never reversed.

Insidiously, these food trends have made their way into our daily eating habits. And the pancreas has been paying the price. Hyperinsulinism will continue to cause obesity, diabetes, and cardiovascular disease.

I hope that this book has made you aware enough of the poor dietary habits in western societies to change the way you eat, whether it is to lose weight or not. If you follow the Montignac Method, I believe you will rediscover your health, reach your ideal weight, and feel better for it.

APPENDIX I:
CRITICISMS OF THE MONTIGNAC METHOD

Because of its unorthodox concept, the Montignac Method has had certain criticisms levelled at it since it first came out in 1987. Journalists, nutritionists, and dieticians have all attacked aspects of it. But many of them never took the time to learn about it properly, and as a result, it has been unduly maligned. I'd like to address the previous and future criticisms that the Montignac Method has and probably will still undergo.

Is the Montignac Method a one-food diet?
Because I concentrate on increasing good carbohydrates into everyone's diet, it does not mean I do not include other foods such as proteins and fats in the Method. In fact, I do. The Montignac Method includes foods from all food groups. It is basically a low-fat, high-fibre diet that is healthy and nutritious. You can see that for yourself after reading the book thoroughly. Is

the Montignac Method based on the food-combining theory of the Hay Method? The Montignac Method is based on discoveries made during the 1970s and 1980s about the metabolism of carbohydrates and lipids, specifically hyperinsulinism, hyperglycemia and the classification of carbohydrates based on their carbohydrate concentration (glycemic index).

The Hay Method, on the other hand, is based on certain tenets of the 19th century. The Hay Method advocated the avoidance of combining certain foods such as carbohydrates and proteins to prevent intoxicating the blood. The goal of the Hay Method (whose principles have been invalidated by modern science) is mostly to cure, or at least prevent, certain diseases of the arteries and digestive problems. It is erroneous, then, to compare the Montignac Method to the Hay Method, even though Hay also advised eating fruit on an empty stomach to avoid digestive problems.

Is the Montignac Method similar to the Atkins diet?
During the 1960s and 1970s, the Atkins diet was very popular. Dr. Atkins claimed that all foods were good to eat except for carbohydrates. He suspected them of causing excess insulin secretion and of being the catalyst to weight gain. But he did not distinguish the difference between carbohydrates and thus banned them all. Unfortunately, the Atkins diet caused its followers to consume too much fat in meats, for example. Consequently, cardiovascular problems increased, and the Atkins diet became known as the "passport to heart attacks.» The Montignac Method is not a "watered-down Atkins diet," as some have charged.

In fact, the Montignac Method is based on consuming a number of low-GI carbohydrates: fruit, vegetables, whole grains, and spaghetti. What's more, I strongly suggest that fat consumption should be carefully monitored (see Chapter 8).

Is there cardiovascular risk in the Montignac Method?

Even though I suggest that on the Montignac Method, you may reasonably eat meat, cheese, and fatty fish, some people have accused the diet of being too fatty. This is not true. I have been careful to discuss all aspects of fats and have clearly explained how to incorporate fats into the diet. This is supported by many experts in the field of cardiology. As a matter of fact, in the preamble and the preface of this book, two cardiologists attest to the benefits of the Montignac Method. Dr. Jean Dumesnil, a cardiologist at the Quebec Heart Institute at Laval University, found that obese men who followed the Montignac Method successfully lowered their lipids and cholesterol[17]. Weight loss—no matter what the diet—automatically leads to a decrease in cholesterol. What's more, I advocate a diet high in fibre, which has been shown to lower cholesterol.

---

17 An important study was published in 2001 by the British Journal of Medicine under the responsibility of the Quebec University. Dr J. DUMESNIL, the leader of this study showed that not only the Montignac diet was the easiest to follow and to get long term results with (compare to others) but it decreases all cardio vascular risk factors.

APPENDIX II:
SPECIAL ADVICE FOR VEGETARIANS

I respect people who have decided not to eat meat because they care for animals. Nevertheless, they must pay close attention to their diets to ensure that they are getting all the nutrients that they require. Vegetarians who do not eat meat, poultry, or fish should consider eating some animal products such as dairy and eggs. They must be knowledgeable about sound nutrition, too. For example, they should know that animal and vegetable proteins are not identical. Some vegetable proteins, for example, are not totally assimilated by the body. Ten grams of protein from lentils will not have the same value as ten grams of egg protein. In fact, one should eat at least one gram of protein per two pounds of body weight. Vegetarians who eat a lot of soy products should know that not all soy foods contain the same amount of protein.

Proteins contained in different soy foods per 3.5 ounces (100g):

- Soy flour: 45 g
- Soy grain: 35 g
- Tofu: 13 g
- Soy germ: 4 g
- Soy sprouts: 1.5 g

Soy milk is low in calcium (42 mg per 4 ounces/113g) compared to cow's milk (120 mg per 4 ounces/113g). In addition, vegetable proteins are lower in essential amino acids (those that the body does not produce on its own), grains are low in lysine and legumes in methionine. It is important, therefore, to combine whole grains, legumes, and nuts on a daily basis. Indeed, many cultures around the world naturally mix grains and legumes: corn and kidney beans in Mexican tortillas, semolina, and chickpeas in Maghrebian couscous, meal and peanuts in black Africa. Eggs, on the other hand, contain a perfect balance of amino acids.

Iron intake needs to be carefully monitored in vegetarians. Iron from vegetable sources is five times harder for the body to assimilate than animal iron. Cheese, eggs, and seaweed will ensure a proper supply of vitamin B12. Properly planned vegetarian meals are healthy, especially in the prevention of heart disease and certain cancers, especially colon and rectal. Children, pregnant women and the elderly should be careful adopting vegetarianism. Consult your doctor first. The Montignac Method is perfectly compatible with vegetarianism. Eating low-GI carbohydrates works well with the requirements of a vegetarian diet.

- whole-wheat bread
- whole-grain bread
- brown rice
- whole-wheat or whole-grain pasta
- lentils
- white and kidney beans
- peas and snow peas
- whole-grain products
- fresh fruits
- nuts
- sugar-free marmalade
- soy products
- chocolate rich in cocoa
- breakfasts of fibre-rich bread or sugar-free cereal with a skim dairy product
- Good carbohydrate dinners three times a week are recommended by the Montignac Method, and vegetarians can eat these meals more frequently. Main courses can include:
- whole-grain rice with tomato sauce
- whole-wheat or whole-grain pasta with a basil, tomato or mushroom sauce
- lentils with onions
- a combination of red and white beans
- peas
- chickpeas
- couscous made from whole semolina
- soy-based products
- grain-based products (whole-wheat crêpes)
- seaweed

These meals can be accompanied by vegetable soup, raw vegetables, or a salad. Desserts can include a dairy product such as
skim cottage cheese or plain yogurt. Vegan diets, which do not
include eggs or dairy, can cause deficiencies. Consult with your
doctor to make sure you are getting all the vitamins, minerals,
and trace elements that you need.

APPENDIX III:
ADVICE FOR WOMEN WHO HAVE TROUBLE LOSING WEIGHT

If, by following the Montignac Method, you are having trouble losing weight, it might be helpful to look at several factors that may be interfering with your success. First of all, be sure you have set the proper goal weight for you. Reread the chapter on calculating your body mass index (BMI). Have you set an unattainable goal based on the influences of glamour magazines and TV images? Also, take into consideration that whereas it may have been easier to lose weight a few years ago, now it is taking a little longer to do so. Make sure that you understand the Montignac Method perfectly. Perhaps you may have misinterpreted the requirements:

- Each week, the Montignac Method recommends eating at least three carbohydrate-rich meals based on whole-grain foods (spaghetti, brown rice, or semolina) or legumes (lentils, white and kidney beans and chickpeas) divided between lunches and dinners. Have you been following that recommendation?

• Protein (60 to 90 g per day, according to your weight) should be eaten on a regular basis. Some people do not follow this recommendation, and that can affect weight loss.

• Do not eat dairy products at each meal. They indeed provide a good source of protein but bear in mind that the whey fraction of the milk/dairy is insulinotropic which increase the weight gain.

• Could you inadvertently be following a low-calorie diet and starving yourself? On the Montignac Method, you lose weight by eating better, not less.

• Are you snacking between meals or drinking alcohol? Doing so compromises weight loss.

Other factors affecting your weight loss could include:

• Hormonal fluctuations, especially during puberty, pregnancy, and menopause.

• Stress can interfere with your weight loss. If you are nervous, grieving, or anxious, your body secretes chemical substances that can prevent weight loss. Learn to manage your stress with relaxation, meditation, or yoga.

• Thyroid problems can block weight loss. Even if you are taking medication and your body has returned to normal, weight loss may still elude you.

• Medications can slow down weight loss: Tranquilizers, anti-depressants, lithium, cortisone, beta blockers, and hormone replacement therapy.

• Former low-calories diet followers must know that once they start the Montignac program the body takes time (weeks and sometimes months) to recover a normal functioning leading to weight loss. Then be patient!

APPENDIX IV:
GETTING ENOUGH PROTEIN

Protein is necessary to replenish that which is lost during cell renewal and to prevent muscle deterioration. Healthy adults should consume about 1g per 2lb. of body weight. So, for a person weighing 155 lb., protein consumption should reach at least 70g per day. However, when a weight-loss program is started, protein intake should be increased: 1.3 to 1.5g per 2lb. of body weight per day. Here's why:

1. First, when you lose weight you also lose muscle mass. To avoid that loss and weakening the body, which occurs when you follow low-calorie diets, it is recommended that you eat more protein than what is required for normal cell renewal.

2. Second, there's some evidence that increased protein intake can actually aid weight loss. Protein-rich foods may make you feel fuller, which will curb your appetite. Digestion of

proteins increases your energy use (thermogenesis). To eliminate the waste left over from protein metabolism, you should drink plenty of liquids throughout the day: 1.5 to 2 quarts.

N.B.: Individuals with kidney problems should consult their doctor before increasing their protein intake. Also, if you're having difficulty losing weight, make sure you're getting enough protein.

GETTING ENOUGH PROTEIN

Animal protein		Vegetable protein	
beef	20 g	rye germ	13 g
veal	20 g	wheat germ	13 g
pork	17 g	barley germ	12 g
mutton	15 g	corn	10 g
cooked ham	18 g	whole-wheat bread	9 g
smoked ham	15 g	whole-wheat pasta	9 g
blood pudding	24 g	white beans	8 g
sausage	25 g	lentils	8 g
chicken	20 g	chickpeas	8 g
one egg	6 g	kidney beans	8 g
fish	30 g	white bread	7 g
Muenster	35 g	wheat semolina	5 g
Gruyère	35 g	white pasta	3 g
brie	20 g	Brown rice	7 g
camembert	20 g	white rice	6 g
cottage cheese	9 g	granola	9 g
yogurt	5 g	Tofu	13g
milk	3.5 g	soy flour	45g
mussels	20 g	doy milk	4 g
shrimp	25 g	Soy germ	4g
soy beans	35 g		
wheat germ	25 g		
oatmeal	13 g		

APPENDIX V:

SUCCESS STORIES AND STUDIES ON THE MONTIGNAC METHOD

Since 1987, we have received hundreds of thousands of letters from people who have successfully followed and are following the Montignac Method. This enormous support has encouraged us to continue to conduct more research into the Method.

We have found that about 85 percent of those who apply the principles of the Montignac Method are able to lose and maintain their ideal weight over the long term.

Only a minority has difficulty losing weight and that's due to unique reasons such as those explained in Appendix III.

Most devotees claim that the Montignac Method is simple and easy to follow. They even tell us that it has restored their pleasure in eating. That's because they see the Montignac Method not as a diet but a lifestyle. Some are happy to remain in Phase I because they feel so good.

Not only have they lost and maintained their weight, but they claim that their gastrointestinal problems have disappeared and that they feel they have attained better physical and psychological health. They no longer complain of fatigue or mid-afternoon slumps. They experience the need for less sleep because it is more refreshing. They also report that they suffer fewer infections.

The following are studies that support the principles of the Montignac Method.

The 1994 French Centre d'Études et d'Information des Vitamines (CEIV) Study

The study's goal was to assess the Montignac Method's nutritional makeup, especially its vitamin content. Patients following the Method kept detailed journals of their meals. This is what the researchers found about the nutritional content of Montignac meals.

They contained on average:

NUTRITIONAL CONTENT OF MONTIGNAC MEALS

Proteins	29.3%
Carbohydrates	39.5%
Fats	31 .2%, including 332 mg of cholesterol per day
Fibre	24.4 g per day
Phosphorus	1,431 mg per day
Magnesium	447 mg
Calcium	1,110 mg
Iron	18.6 mg
Sodium	1,643 mg
Potassium	3,465 mg
Vitamin C	198 mg
Vitamin B1	2.6 mg
Vitamin B2	3.1 mg
Vitamin B6	1.8 mg
Vitamin PP	24 mg
Vitamin E	10.1 mg
Vitamin D	1.4 mg
Vitamin A	6,939 IU
Vitamin B9	509 mg
Beta-carotene	6,400 mg

According to this study, the Montignac Method is among the best of the weight-loss diets in terms of vitamins and mineral intake. In addition, fat content was 31.2 percent, falling well within current nutritional guidelines.

Studies by Drs. Caupin and Robert (1994)

Some 150 women from the ages of 18 to 68 years of age were studied at the Institut Vitalité et Nutrition in Paris. They were divided into three groups based on their BMI (see Chapter 12):

- 32 women had a BMI less than 24
- 80 women had a BMI between 24 and 29
- 38 women had a BMI greater than 29

RESULTS AT THE END OF FOUR MONTHS:

BMI	Average weight loss	Percentage of weight lost	Drop in BMI	Percentage of drop in BMI
<24	−5.47 kg	−8.81%	−2.11	−9.2%
24-29	−8.71 kg	−11.86%	−3.24	−11.85%
>29	−13.37 kg	−1 4.42%	−5.09	−4.55%

RESULTS AT THE END OF ONE YEAR:

BMI	Average weight loss	Percentage of weight lost	Drop in BMI	Percentage of drop in BMI
<24	−4.38 kg	−6.74%	−1.76	−7.9%
24-29	−8.14 kg	−1 0.41%	−3.00	−10.9%
>29	−18.46 kg	−1 9.77%	−6.96	−20.22%

These women were well aware of the principles of the Montignac Method, either because they had read the book or were taught by their family doctors.

Comments

• The women whose BMI was less than 24 (a normal build for a woman 1.65 m tall or 5'5" and weighing 60 kg or 132 lb.) wanted to be thinner than they were. Nevertheless, after four months, they did achieve an average weight loss of about 5.5 kg (12 lb.). A year later, they had only regained 1 kg (2.2 lb.).

• The women whose BMI was between 24 and 29, which indicates an excess of only a few pounds (a woman 1.65 m or 5'5" tall and weighing 70 kg, about 155 lb., has a BMI of 27), lost an average of 8.7 kg or about 19 lb., over four months. They reached their ideal weight and maintained that weight within 600 g for a year.

• The group whose BMI was between 30 and 40, which is considered obese, lost an average of 13.4 kg (30 lb.). At the end of one year, the average weight loss was 18.5 kg (about 40 lb.).

Canadian study by profs. Dumesnil and Tremblay

Cardiologist Jean Dumesnil at the Quebec Heart Institute in Quebec City was overweight and was experiencing difficulty shedding his excess pounds. Professor Tremblay, a nutritionist and colleague, suggested he try the Montignac Method. When Dumesnil lost 21 kg (about 46 lb.), Tremblay was so intrigued that in 1997 they began a study to determine the reason for Dumesnil's success. The researchers compared the effects of three diets in men in their late 40s with BMIs of 28 and an average weight of 103 kg (225 lb.). On all three diets, the participants could eat as much as they wanted. Diet 2 Group (Montignac Method) only ate low-GI carbohydrates.

COMPARED EFFECTS OF THREE DIETS

	Diet 1	Diet 2 (Montignac)	Diet 3
Proteins	15%	31%	16%
Fats	30%	32%	30%
Carbohydrates	55%	37%	54%

• Diet 1, which comprised classic dieting advice, given by the AHA (American Hart Association). Actually this diet caused a slight weight gain and showed non significant decrease for the cardio-vascular risk factors.

• Diet 2, the Montignac Method, curbed appetites while at the same time satisfied the participants. Low-GI carbohydrates and high-protein content contributed to this success. The average weight loss was 2.4 percent. One participant who weighed 102 kg (225 lb.) lost as much as 3.2 kg (6.5 lb.) in one week. What's more, men on the Montignac Method experienced a reduction in cardiovascular risks. For instance, the triglycerids dropped incredibly by 35%.

• Diet 3, which had the same calorie content as Diet 2, but a different nutritional content, only resulted in a 1.7 percent weight loss.

This Canadian study was published in the "British Journal of Nutrition" in November 2001. In the summer of 1999, two large epidemiological studies conducted in the United States over a 12-year period by Professor Walter Willett of Harvard University's School of Public Health was officially published.

These studies will show that the consumption of high-GI carbohydrates leads to obesity, diabetes, and heart disease. Dr. Willett also disagrees with the standard recommendations to consume more carbohydrates and fewer fats. He believes that those recommendations are largely responsible for the prevalence of obesity in the American population.

APPENDIX VI:
RECIPES

The purpose of this book is not to offer you a cookbook filled
with impressive recipes. For that there are already a number of
Montignac cookbooks available in bookstores. But if you have
understood and are applying basic dietary principles to meet the
goals you've set yourself, you should be able to create your own
recipes or, at the very least, adapt existing ones.

The Montignac dietary principles are applied to choosing foods
and cooking methods as follows:

• Eliminate all high-GI carbohydrates (sugars, starches) which
have the potential of elevating glycemic levels, in particular:

  - Sugar (sucrose)
  - White flour
  - Potatoes

- Carrots (cooked, not raw)
- Corn
- White rice (with the exception of Basmati)
- Oriental noodles, macaroni, ravioli

• Include low-GI carbohydrates, which encourage weight loss, such as:

- Lentils
- Dry beans
- Peas
- Chickpeas
- Green vegetables (lettuce, broccoli, cabbage, green beans, spinach, eggplant, peppers, tomatoes, zucchini)
- Whole grains (unrefined flours)
- fruit

• Eliminate bad fats and replace with good fats.

• Avoid:

- Cooked butter (such as clarified butter)
- Processed oils
- Palm oil
- Lard
- Margarine

- Include:

  - Olive oil
  - Goose fat
  - Duck fat
  - Sunflower oil
  - Canola oil

- Choose fish and poultry over red meat.

- Avoid cooking at high temperatures, especially frying.

- Apply these principles in everyday food preparation as follows:

  -Entrées: Avoid foods made with white flour and butter (puff pastry, quiche, pancakes, pie crusts, canapes, croutons).

  - Main dishes: Avoid breaded foods and use grated Parmesan cheese instead of bread crumbs if needed, avoid all sauces made with butter and especially wheat flour, using lentil or chickpea flour instead, and keep this in mind when preparing fish, meat and poultry dishes. Use any kind of cheese (except processed) and yogurt.

  - Desserts: They should not contain flour, butter or sugar, but be made with fruit mousses, eggs, low-fat cream cheese or cottage cheese, ground almonds and hazelnuts, bittersweet chocolate (70 percent cocoa bean content) and fructose. Wine may also be used.

BUCKWHEAT PANCAKES
(Makes 2 pancakes)

1/4 cup (75 ml) buckwheat flour
1 Tbsp (15 ml) wheat germ
1/4 cup (75 ml) water
1 tsp (5 ml) olive oil

• Mix dry ingredients. Gradually add water and mix to a smooth batter. Let sit for about 5 minutes.

• Over medium heat, heat a very lightly oiled non-stick frying pan, add half the batter, tilting the pan to cover. Cook, turning once.

• Garnish with stewed fruit, sugar-free jam, or non-fat cheese.

BEAN SOUP
(Serves 4)

14 oz(400g) mixed, dry beans
1 small onion
2 cloves garlic, peeled and minced
4 celery sticks
1/2 green bell pepper
1/2 red bell pepper
1 tbsp (15 ml) olive oil
1/4 cup (75 ml) hulled barley
4 cups (1 L) water
1 cup (250 ml) canned tomatoes, drained
2 tbsp (30 ml) tamari (pure soy sauce)
1 bay leaf
1/2 tsp (2 ml) dried oregano
1/2 tsp (2 ml) dried basil
1/4 tsp (1 ml) dried tarragon
1 tbsp (15 ml) chopped fresh parsley

• Soak beans overnight. Rinse. Dice onion, celery, and peppers. In a saucepan, over medium heat, heat olive oil. Add diced vegetables and garlic, and sauté 5 minutes.

• Add barley, water, and beans. Let simmer 30 minutes.

• Add tomatoes, tamari, bay leaf, oregano, basil, tarragon, and parsley. Simmer 5-10 minutes more.

FLOURLESS SOUFFLÉ
(Serves 4-5)

3/4 lb (300 g) quark-style cheese (0% fat)
6 oz (150g) grated Gruyère cheese
4 egg yolks
Salt and pepper
4 egg whites

- Pre-heat oven to 220°C (425°F).

- Mix the cheeses into egg yolks. Add salt and pepper to taste.

- Beat egg white until stiff. Fold into cheese mixture. Pour into a 20 cm (8 in.) soufflé dish.

- Bake at 220°C (425°F) 30 minutes until golden.

- Serve immediately.

Option: Add to soufflé mixture 100 g (3 oz) lean ham or 10 puréed button mushrooms.

TUNA GELATINE MOUSSE
(Serves 6-8)

1 envelope (15 ml/1 tbsp) unsweetened gelatine
1 cup (250 ml) dry white wine
2 cans (170g/6 oz each) tuna packed in water
1 tsp (5 ml) mustard
3 tbsp (45 ml) olive oil
1 tbsp (45 ml) fresh chopped parsley
1 tsp (5 ml) salt
Pepper
1 tbsp (15 ml) wine vinegar
1/2 cup (125 ml) fresh white cheese, such as quark or fromage frais
Garnish: Sliced hard-cooked eggs, lettuce, sliced tomatoes, parsley

• In a small mixing bowl, dissolve gelatine in 45 ml (3 tbsp) white wine. Bring rest of the wine to boil and pour over gelatine. Mix well and let cool.

• Drain tuna and flake.

• Mix together mustard, olive oil, parsley, salt, pepper and vinegar.

• When gelatine is lukewarm, add tuna and cheese, and mix well.

• Pour into a lightly oiled cake mould and let set in refrigerator 2-3 hours.

• Turn onto a platter lined with lettuce leaves, and garnish with tomato, egg, and parsley. Service with plain or herbed mayonnaise.

TOMATO TART
(Serves 4)

1 lb. (500 g) cherry tomatoes
2 tbsp (30 ml) olive oil
4 fresh eggs
1 3/4 cups (400 ml) 15% fat cream
2 tbsp (30 ml) chopped fresh basil
Salt, black pepper, cayenne

• In an ovenproof dish, place tomatoes, drizzle with olive oil and bake in 150°C (300°F) oven 30 minutes.

• In a mixing bowl, beat eggs, add cream and basil, season with salt, pepper, and cayenne.

• Divide mixture into 4 10-cm (4-in.) ramekins. Top with tomatoes and bake 15 minutes.

• Serve hot or cold with an entrée.

LEGUME PÂTÉ
(Makes 500 ml/2 cups)

1 can pinto beans, rinsed and drained
1/2 of a 396 ml/14 oz can lentils, rinsed and drained
3 tbsp (45 ml) chopped onion
2 tbsp (30 ml) lemon juice
1 tbsp (15 ml) parsley
1 tsp (5 ml) powdered vegetable broth
1/2 tsp (1 ml) ground pepper
1/2 garlic clove, peeled and minced

• Process all the ingredients in a food processor until smooth.
Place in a bowl and refrigerate 1 hour.

Can be served as a dip, with vegetables or whole-wheat crackers.

ORANGE BROCCOLI
(Serves 4)

1 head broccoli
Zest of 1 orange
1 tsp (5 ml) olive oil
Salt and pepper

• Separate broccoli into spears; place in a saucepan with 2.5 cm (1 in.) water. Bring to boil and cook 2 minutes. Add zest, cover, and cook 2 minutes more.

• Drain broccoli, drizzle with olive oil, season with salt and pepper.

• Serve hot.

ZUCCHINI TOMATO CASSEROLE
(Serves 8)

6 zucchini
6 tomatoes
1 1/4 cups (300 ml) 15% fat cream
6 eggs
3 tbsp (45 ml) chopped fresh basil
2 tbsp (30 ml) chopped fresh parsley
Pinch nutmeg
Pinch cayenne
1 tbsp (15 ml) olive oil
2 cloves garlic, peeled and crushed
Salt and pepper

• Wash and slice zucchini and tomatoes.

• In a bowl, mix cream, eggs, herbs, nutmeg, cayenne, salt, and pepper.

• Lightly oil an ovenproof dish. Place sliced zucchini and tomatoes in alternate layers. Pour olive oil over, season with salt and pepper, and bake at 180°C (350°F) for 20 minutes.

• Remove casserole, pour in egg mixture. Bake 30-35 minutes more. Serve hot.

CAULIFLOWER LOAF
(Serves 8-10)

1 head cauliflower, separated into florets
3 oz (100 g) quark or other low-fat cream cheese
1/2 cup (125 ml) powdered milk, mixed with a little water to a thick, smooth consistency
6 eggs
Salt and pepper

• Cook cauliflower in salted water 5 minutes and drain. (It should still be crunchy.)

• Purée in food processor; add cheese, milk, eggs, salt and pepper.
 Mix well and transfer to a greased cake mould.

• Place cake mould in a shallow pan of water and bake in 200°C (400°F) oven 1 hour.

• Remove from oven, let sit 15 minutes, then unmould.

• Serve hot or warm with a tomato coulis.

TOMATO COULIS
(Makes 500 ml/2 cups)

1 tbsp (15 ml) olive oil
1 clove garlic, peeled and crushed
28 oz (800g) can tomatoes
1 tsp (5 ml) dried herbs (oregano, basic, tarragon)
Salt and pepper

- In a sauté pan, heat olive oil; add garlic and cook 30 seconds. Add tomatoes and seasonings immediately, and simmer 15 minutes.

- Process in blender or food processor to a smooth purée.

- Serve with vegetables, whole grains, or legumes.

RED-PEPPER COULIS
(Makes 375 ml/1 $^{1/2}$ cups)

1 tbsp (15 ml) olive oil
1 garlic clove, peeled and minced
1 shallot, chopped
2 red peppers
3/4 cup (200 ml) defatted chicken broth
Salt and pepper
Pinch of cayenne

• In a small saucepan, over low heat, heat oil and cook shallot, 1 minute.

• Seed and dice peppers, and add to shallot. Mix and cook 2 minutes.

• Add broth and simmer 3 minutes.

• Process in blender to smooth consistency. Season.

• Serve with vegetables, whole grains, or legumes.

SPAGHETTI WITH EGGPLANT &
SWEET AND SOUR TOMATO SAUCE

(Serves 4)

2 medium tomatoes
1 onion
2 small or 1 medium eggplant
1/4 cup (60 ml) olive oil
1 bouquet garni
2 tbsp (30 ml) chopped fresh basil
Salt, black pepper, cayenne
3 tbsp (45 ml) balsamic vinegar
14 oz (400 g) spaghetti

- Parboil tomatoes 1 minute. Peel, remove seeds, and chop.

- Peel and finely chop onion. Wash and dice eggplant.

- In a sauté pan, cook onion in 1 tbsp oil until soft. Add tomatoes, bouquet garni, basil, salt, pepper, and cayenne, and cook 15 minutes.

- Add balsamic vinegar, remove from heat, and remove bouquet garni.

- In a separate pan, sauté eggplant in the rest of the oil. Season, cook 6-7 minutes, and add to tomato sauce.

- Cook spaghetti in boiling salted water until *al dente*. Drain. Add sauce, toss, and adjust seasoning.

SUCCULENT RICE
(Makes 500 ml/2 cups)

1 tbsp (15 ml) olive oil
1 tsp (5 ml) ground cumin
3 cloves
1 cinnamon stick (or 1 ml/1 tsp ground)
1 cup (250 ml) Basmati rice
2 cups (500 ml) vegetable broth
2 bay leaves

• In a saucepan, over medium heat, heat oil. Add cumin, cloves, and cinnamon. Stir about 1 minute.

• Add rice and stir. Add broth and bay leaves. Cover, reduce heat and simmer 20 minutes, or until rice has absorbed the liquid.

• Remove bay leaves, cinnamon stick, and cloves.

• Garnish with sunflower seeds, nuts, or legumes, and serve.

COD PÂTÉ
(Serves 5)

2 lb (1 kg) cod fillets
2 cups (500 ml) court-bouillon or vegetable broth
2 lemons
1 can (156 ml / 5 1/2-oz) tomato paste
Salt and pepper

• Poach the cod in barely simmering court-bouillon. Add juice and zest of lemons, and let simmer 20 minutes more.

• Remove cod and drain well, pressing all liquid out with your hands. Cut into large pieces.

• Place in a lightly greased cake tin or soufflé dish.

• Beat the eggs, add tomato paste, salt, and pepper, and pour over the cod.

• Bake in a 150°C (325°F) oven 30 minutes.

• Refrigerate at least 6 hours or overnight. Turn onto a serving dish and serve cold with mayonnaise.

MAYONNAISE
(Makes 250 ml/1 cup)

1 egg
1 tsp (5 ml) (Dijon) mustard
1 tsp (5 ml) lemon juice
1/2 tsp (2 ml) salt
1 cup (250 ml) olive oil

• In a blender, place egg, mustard, lemon juice and salt, and process 30 seconds. With the blender running, add oil in a thin, steady stream through the opening in the lid.

• Mayonnaise is done when thick and creamy.

• Store in refrigerator.

• To "stretch" the mayonnaise, add one beaten egg white.

SPICY FISH
(Serves 5)

4 sole fillets, 125 g (4 oz) each
1 tsp (5 ml) garlic powder
1 tsp (5 ml) paprika
1 tsp (5 ml) onion powder
1/2 tsp (2 ml) oregano
1/2 tsp (2 ml) thyme
1/2 tsp (2 ml) salt
1/4 tsp (1 ml) white pepper
1/4 tsp (1 ml) black pepper
1/4 tsp (1 ml) cayenne
10 ml (2 tsp) olive oil

• In a shallow dish, mix seasonings and coat fillets.

• In a non-stick skillet, over medium heat, heat a little oil. Add fillets and cook 2-3 minutes on each side, until seasonings are golden and fish starts to separate.

• Serve with Tomato Coulis (see page 215) or Red-Pepper Coulis (see page 216).

BLUEBERRY BLANCMANGE
(Serves 4)

1 envelope (15 ml/1 tbsp) unsweetened gelatine or agar agar
1/3 cup (100 ml) white wine
1 tsp (5 ml) vanilla extract
1 cup (250 ml) 15% cream
1/4 cup (60 ml) fructose
8 oz (250 g) 0% quark or other non-fat cream cheese
2 cups (500 ml) blueberries
2 tbsp (30 ml) sugar-free blueberry jelly
1/2 cup (125 ml) port
Juice of 1 orange

• Stir gelatine into 45 mm (3 tbsp) cold water. In a sauce-pan, heat the wine, add gelatine, and dissolve. Let cool; stir in vanilla.

• Whip the cream.

• Combine 45 ml (3 tbsp) of the fructose with cheese, whipped cream, and wine. Spoon some of the mixture into 4 ramekins, and refrigerate at least 3 hours.

• In a saucepan, bring to boil blueberries, blueberry jelly, and port. With a slotted spoon, remove berries. Add orange juice and fructose to the mixture and continue cooking until reduced to a syrup consistency. Pour syrup over the berries.

• To serve, unmold ramekins onto individual plates, and pour blueberry sauce over.

LIME MOUSSE
(Serves 4)

2 eggs
2 tbsp (30 g) fructose
Juice of 2 fresh limes
Pinch salt
1 tbsp (15 ml) chopped fresh mint
14 oz (400 g) non-fat cream cheese or quark

• Separate the eggs. Beat yolks with fructose; when mixture turns white, add lime juice.

• Add pinch of salt to egg whites and beat until stiff; gently fold into yolk mixture. Fold in mint and cheese.

• Divide mixture into 4 dessert bowls and refrigerate at least 4 hours.

• Serve alone or with your choice of fresh berries.

STRAWBERRY ICE
(Serves 8-10)

1 lb (500 g) strawberries
5 egg whites
3 oz (100 g) non-fat cream cheese or quark
3 tbsp (45 ml) fructose
2 tbsp (30 ml) lemon juice
For the sauce:
10 oz (300 g) strawberries
1 tbsp (15 ml) fructose
Juice of 1/2 lemon

• Purée strawberries in a blender or using an electric beater. Beat egg whites until stiff.

• Into puréed strawberries, fold egg whites, cheese and fructose until well blended and creamy. Add lemon juice. Pour mixture into a greased cake mould.

• Freeze 6-7 hours. Remove from freezer 1/2 hour before serving. Unmold; run lukewarm water over mould if necessary.

To make the sauce:

• Purée all ingredients in a blender.

• To serve, spoon sauce over and garnish with fresh strawberry halves.

RASPBERRY BAVAROISE
(Serves 5-6)

1 envelope (15 ml/1 tbsp) unsweetened gelatine or agar agar
4 egg yolks
1 1/4 cup (300 ml) milk
2 cups (500 ml) raspberries
3 tbsp (45 ml) fructose
For the sauce:
1 1/2 cup (375 ml) raspberries
Juice of 1 lemon
1 tsp(5 ml) fructose

• Dissolve gelatine in 45 ml (3 tbsp) cold water.

• In a saucepan, beat egg yolks, add milk, and stir over low heat until mixture thickens enough to cover back of a spoon. Remove from heat.

• Purée raspberries in a blender; add fructose.

• Stir gelatine into warm egg yolk mixture; add raspberry purée and stir.

• Pour into a lightly greased bavaroise mould and refrigerate at least 12 hours, until bavaroise is set.

To make the sauce:

• Purée ingredients in a blender, and refrigerate until needed.

• Spoon onto dishes or serve on the side.

CHOCOLATE MOUSSE
(Serves 8)

1 lb (500 g) bittersweet chocolate (70% cocoa bean)
1/2 cup (125 ml) strong black coffee
1/4 cup (75 ml) rum
Zest of 1 orange
8 large eggs
Pinch of salt

• Break the chocolate into pieces and place in double boiler along with the coffee and rum. Melt over low heat, stirring now and then with a spatula. If consistency is too thick, add a little water. As soon as the chocolate has completely melted into a thick, unctuous liquid, remove pan from heat and let cool.

• Mix half the zest into the mixture.

• Separate eggs, playing yolks in one bowl and the white in another. Add a pinch of salt to egg white and beat until stiff.

• Pour chocolate mixture into bowl containing the egg yolks. Mix thoroughly until well blended. Transfer into bowl containing egg whites, and fold in gently until completely blended. Make sure there are no unmixed pieces of chocolate or egg whites at the bottom of the bowl. Transfer mousse to a serving bowl or individual bowls, and refrigerate at least 6 hours, preferably overnight. Sprinkle with remaining orange zest.

MICHEL MONTIGNAC PRODUCTS

FOR NUTRITIOUS GOURMET EATING

Michel Montignac has created an exclusive line of food products specially for his dietary method. All are rich in fibre, with no added sugar, and made with whole-wheat flour. They all conform to the low GI. No colourings, additives, or modified starches are used. Among these are grain products such as organic whole-wheat breads, chocolate containing 85 percent cocoa bean, and non-sugar jam. Michel Montignac products are available in several countries.

Official website: **www.montignac.com**

Shop online: **www.montignac-shop.com**

Coaching online: **www.methode-montignac.com**

GLOSSARY

Adipose cells: Another term for fat cells.

Amino acids: Organic molecules made up primarily of carbon nitrogen, hydrogen, and oxygen, whose chemical combination creates a protein.

Antioxidants: Prevent oxidization, fight free radicals that circulate in the body. Beta-carotene and vitamins C and E are known as the antioxidant vitamins.

Body mass index (BMI): A way of measuring obesity. Consists of determining the Quetelet index, also known as body mass index. It is arrived at by dividing body weight in kilograms by height in square metres. It allows classification of adults age 20-65 into one of five categories (see Chapter 12).

Bolting: process by which flour is refined, during which bran is removed.

Carbohydrate: Another term for glucide.

Cholesterolemia: Concentration of cholesterol in the blood.

Chronobiology: Assimilation of food by the body, which varies depending on the time of day or even season.

Dextrose: Another term for glucose. Found in fruit and in the blood after digestion of glucides.

Enzymes: Complex proteins produced by living cells that catalyze specific biochemical reactions at body temperatures. For example, lipase is an enzyme that accelerates the breakdown of proteins and enables the blood to carry them to the cells.

Essential fatty acids: Fatty acids not manufactured by the body, which have to be obtained through food. Needed for absorption of fat-soluble vitamins, i.e., vitamins that dissolve in fats, such as A, D, E, K. (NOTE: Also known as linoleic acid and alphalimonelic acid. Linoleic acid is a liquid unsaturated fatty acid).

Extrusion: Process by which dough is forced out of machine at high pressure. This creates a film around thin pasta like spaghetti, and limits the gelatinization of starch during cooking.

Fibre: Undigestible complex glucides found in vegetables. It increases the volume of ingested food and decreases the amount of time in the intestines.

Free radicals: Wastes in the body that can contribute to cell and genetic damage. They can occur in two ways: through environmental pollution, tobacco, alcohol, or drugs, or through normal reactions of the body. They contribute to the acceleration of the aging process and are an important factor in causing serious illnesses (cataracts, hypertension, cancer).

Fructose: Naturally occurring simple glucide found in fruit (2 to 7 percent), honey (40 percent) and other foods. It is one and a half times sweeter than ordinary sugar.

Glucagon: Hormone produced by the pancreas; increases sugar content of blood.

Glucides: Also called "carbohydrates" or "sugars." Composed of carbon and oxygen. They include simple glucides (glucose, fructose, galactose), double glucides (sucrose, maltose, lactose) and starch, a complex, unsweet glucide.

Glucose: Simple glucide found in the blood, and a source of energy for the body.

Glycemia: Level of glucose (sugar) in the blood.

Glycemic index (GI): Measurement of glucidic foods, the amount of glucose entering the blood after the ingestion of sugar; the higher the glycemic index of a food, the more the food increases sugar in the blood, thus increasing the secretion of insulin.

Glycemic outcome: Average increase of glycemia (level of sugar in the blood) after a meal, depending on the quantity and quality of glucides consumed, as well as the protein and fibre eaten at the same time.

Hormones: Chemicals secreted by a gland, which, when released in the blood, produce an effect on the activity of cells remote from their point of origin.

Hydrogenation: Commercial process that permits hardening of oils (i.e., shortening, margarine). The process alters the fatty acids, which become saturated or unsaturated (transfatty acids).

Hypercholesterolemia: High level of cholesterol in the blood.

Hyperglycemia: High level of glucose in the blood.

Hyperinsulinism: Overproduction of insulin by the pancreas.

Hyperplasia: Abnormal or unusual increase in the elements composing tissue cells.

Hypoglycemia: Abnormal decrease of glucose in the blood.

Insulin: Hormone released by the pancreas that lowers the level of glucose in the blood.

Insulinemia: Abnormally high level of insulin in the blood.

Insulin resistance: The body's reaction to insulin. When hyperglycemic, the body's sensitivity to insulin decreases, and the body needs more and more insulin to reduce the glycemia to normal levels.

Limiting factor: Vegetable proteins (rice, red beans) that contain only partial essential amino acids, and, according to the theory of complementary foods, must be combined with other foods to get the full complement of amino acids. For example, grains are weak in lysine while legumes are rich in them. A meal that includes both grains and legumes constitutes a good combination (i.e., vegetarian chili served with brown rice).

Lipids: Organic substances containing carbon, hydrogen, and oxygen. Often classified under fatty substances, fats, and fatty.

Metabolism: Basal metabolism maintains the essential functions of our bodies (breathing, maintaining body temperature, etc.), which are in fact automatic. Metabolism, in its larger sense, handles the calories we consume and the calories we burn. This includes basal metabolism, energy that is burned through physical activity and the work of the digestive system (transformation of food into energy that the body can use).

Mineral salts: Essential for the body in minimal quantities (calcium, potassium, sodium, etc.). Combined with other nutrients, they are necessary to the efficient functioning of the body.

Modified starch: Commercially treated, which modifies the nutritional content, therefore no longer natural. It is found in a multitude of products (sauces, desserts, salad dressings, sour cream, peanut butter, baby foods).

Monounsaturated fatty acids: Fatty acids containing a single saturated chemical bond. They liquefy at room temperature and harden at 4°C.

Nutrients: Nutritive substances used by the body to grow, to maintain, and repair cells. The major nutrients are protein, glucides and lipids.

Oleaginous plants: Cultivated for their seeds or fruit rich in lipids, from which oils are extracted for consumption or commercial purposes (soy, walnut, sunflower).

Osteomalacia: Progressive softening (demineralization) of the bones caused by the lack of vitamin D, needed for absorption of phosphorus and calcium. It causes pain in the bones and can precipitate fractures.

Osteoporosis: Decrease in bone mass resulting from disturbance of nutrition and mineral metabolism. Causes fractures.

Oxidization: Chemical reaction through which oxygen loses its original structure by combining with another substance and so undergoing a chemical change. Oxidization causes oil to go rancid.

Pancreas: Gland situated behind the stomach, between the spleen and the duodenum. Releases endocrine secretions (insulin and glucagon) and exocrine (digestive enzymes).

Photo-sensitivity: Fear of light because of the discomfort, even pain, it creates.

Polyphenols: Strong antioxidants that help neutralize free radicals. Found in red and blue pigmented fruit such as blueberries, and wines (especially red wines).

Polyunsaturated fatty acids: Fatty acids rich in unsaturated chemical bonds. Usually liquid at room temperature.

Processed Foods: Refining foods for longer shelf life. This process, however, results in the loss of much of the foods' nutritive value (vitamins and minerals).

Protein: Complex combination of amino acids; main constituant of cells.

Saturated fatty acids: Contain the maximum number of carbon atoms in a single chemical bond. Usually of animal origin and remain solid at room temperature.

Starch: Type of glucide from vegetables (grains, legumes, tubers [potatoes, yams, Jerusalem artichokes]) as well as some fruits.

Sucrose: Powdered or in cubes from beets or sugar cane.

Sugars: Term misused in current language to describe glucides, as in "slow sugars" and "fast sugars." The expression "level of sugar in the blood" describes the level of blood glucose (glycemia).

Sweeteners: Artificial sugars with highly concentrated sweetness, used to replace sugar because of their zero-calorie content. Artificial sweeteners include cyclamate, saccharine and aspartame.

Trace elements: Minerals occurring in tiny quantities in the body (iron, zinc, iodine, copper, etc.) to fortify our natural defenses. They allow the body to utilize the basic materials: protein, glucide, and lipids.

Transfatty acids: Unsaturated fatty acids, which are modified. They tend to block the arteries, and raise cholesterol and triglyceride levels of the blood. Found mainly in commercially prepared foods: cookies, crackers, pastries, fried foods, and breaded fish.

Triglycerides: Fatty substances found in the blood, caused by the fats we consume, especially saturated fatty acids and glucides.

Vitamins: Very important organic compounds, of which even a trace is enough to ensure growth and maintenance of the body. Vitamins are known by one letter (A, C, D, E, K and the B group).

BIBLIOGRAPHY

PROTEINS

APFELBAUM M., FORRAT C., NILLUS P., *Diététique et nutrition*, Ed. Masson 1989.

BOURRE J.-M., *De l'animal à l'assiette*, Ed. Odile Jacob, 1993.

BRINGER J., RICHARD J.-L., MIROUZE J., *Évaluation de l'état nutritionnel protéique*, Rev. Prat. 1985, 35, 3, 17-22.

CHELTIEL J.C., *Protéines alimentaires*, Ed, Tech et Doc Lavoisier, 1985.

RUASSE J.P., *Les composants de la matière vivante*, Ed. L'indispensable en nutrition, 1988.

RUASSE J.P., *Des protides, pourquoi, combien?*, Ed. L'indispensable en nutrition, 1987.

CARBOHYDRATES

ANDERSON J.W., *Hypocholesterolemic effects of oat and bean products*, Am. J. Clin. Nutr., 1988, 48, 749-753.

ANDERSON J.W., *Serum lipid response of hypercholesterolemic men to single and divided doses of canned beans*, Eur. J. Clin. Nutr. 1990, 51, 1013-1019.

AUBERT C., *L'assiette aux céréales*, Ed. Terre vivante, 1991.

BANTLE J.P, LAINE D.C., *Post prandial glucose and insulin responses to meals containing different carbohydrates in normal and diabetic subjets*, New Engl. J. Med. 1983, 309, 7-12.

BORNET F., *Place des glucides simples et des produits amylacés dans l'alimentation des diabétiques en 1985*, Fondation

RONAC, Paris.

BROWN, *Coronary heart disease and the consumption of diet high in wheat and other grains*, Am. J. Clin. Nutr., 1985, 41, 1163-117 1.

CALET C., *Les légumes secs, apport protidique*, Cah. Nutr. Diet., 1992, XXVII, 2, 99-108.

CHEW I., *Application of glycemic index to mixed meals*, Am. J. Clin. Nutr., 1988, 47, 53-56.

CRAPO P.A., *Plasma glucose and insulin responses to orally administered simple and complex carbohydrates*, Diabetes, 1976, 25, 74 1-747.

CRAPO P.A., *Post prandial plasma glucose and insulin response to different complex carbohydrates*, Diabetes, 1977, 26, 1178- 1183.

CRAPO P.A., *Comparison of serum glucose-insulin and glucagon responses to different types of carbohydrates in non insulin dependant diabetic patients*, Am J. Clin. Nutr., 1981, 34, 84-90.

DANQUECHIN-DORVAL E., *Rôle de la phase gastrique de la digestion sur la biodisponibilité des hydrates de carbone et leurs effets métaboliques*, Journées de diabétologie de l'Hôtel-Dieu, 1975.

DESJEUX J.F., *Glycémie, insuline et acides gras dans le plasma d'adolescents sains après ingestion de bananes*, Med. et Nutr., 1982, 18, 2, 127-130.

FEWKES D.W., *Sucrose-Science Progress*, 1971, 59, 25, 39.

FITZ-HENRY A., *In vitro and in vivo rates of carbohydrate digestion in Aboriginal bushfoods and contemporary Western foods* (Colloque 1982 de l'Université de Sydney).

GABREAU T., LEBLANC H., *Les modifications de la vitesse d'absorption des glucides*, Med. et Nutr., 1983, XIX, 6, 447-449.

GUILLAUSSEAU P.J, GUILLAUSSEAU-SCHOLER C., *Effet hyperglycémiant des aliments*, Gaz. Med. Fr., 1989, 96, 30, 61-63.

HEATON K.W., *Particule size of wheat, maïze and oat test meals: effects on plasma glucose and insulin responses and on the rate of starch digestion in vitro*, Am. J. Clin. Nutr., 1988, 47, 675-682.

HODORA D., *Glucides simples, glucides complexes et glucides indigestibles*, Gaz. Med. Fr., 1981, 88, 37, 5, 255-259.

JENKINS D.J.A., *Glycemic index of foods: a physiological basis for carbohydrates exchange*, Am. J. Clin. Nutr., 1981, 34, 362- 366.

JENKINS D.J.A., *Dietary carbohydrates and their glycemic responses*, J.A.M.A., 1984, 2, 388-391.

JENKINS D. J.A., *Wholemeal versus whole grain breads: proportion of whole or cracked grains and the glycemic response*, Br. Med. J., 1988, 297, 958-960.

JIAN R., *La vidange d'un repas ordinaire chez l'homme : étude par la méthode radio-isotopique*, Nouv. Presse Med., 1979, 8, 667-671.

KERIN O'DEA, *Physical factor influencing post prandial glucose and insulin responses to starch*, Am. J. Clin. Nutr., 1980, 33, 760-765.

MESSING B., *Sucre et nutrition*, Ed. Doin, 1992.

NOUROT J., *Relationship between the rate of gastric emptying and glucose insulin responses to starchy food in young healthy adults*, Am. J. Clin. Nutr., 1988, 48, 1035-1040.

NATHAN D., *Ice-cream in the diet of insulin-dependant diabetic patients*, J.A.M.A., 1984, 251, 21, 2825-2827.

NICOLAIDIS S., *Mode d'action des substances de goût sucré sur le métabolisme et sur la prise alimentaire. Les sucres dans l'alimentation*, Cool. Sc. Fond. Fr. Nutr., 1981.

O'DONNEL L.J.D., *Size of flour particles and its relation to glycemia, imulinaemia and caloric disease*, Br. Med. J., 17 June 1984, 298, 115-116.

PICHARD P., *Les céréales énergétiques*, Ed. M.A., 1992.

PIVETAUD J., PACCALIN J., *Mais mangez donc des légumineuses!*, Diététique et Médecine, 1993, n° 4, 149-153.

REAVEN C., *Effects of source of dietary carbohydrates on plasma glucose and insulin to test meals in normal subjects.* Am. J. Clin. Nutr., 1980, 33, 1279-1283.

ROUX E., *Index glycémique.* Gaz. Med. Fr., 1988, 95, 18, 77-78.

RUASSE J.P., *Des glucides, pourquoi, comment ?*, Coll. L'indispensable en nutrition.

SCHLIENGER J.L., *Signification d'une courbe d'hyperglycémie orale plate, comparaison avec un repas d'épreuve*, Nouv. Pr. Med., 1982, 52, 3856-3857.

SCHWEITZER T.F., *Nutrients excreted in ileostomy effluents after consumption of mixed diet with beans and potatoes*, Eur. J. Clin. Nutr., 1990, 44, 567-575.

SLAMA G., *Correlation between the nature of amount of carbohydrates in intake and insulin delivery by the artificial pancreas in 24 insulino-dependant diabetics*, 1981, 30, 101-105.

SLAMA G., *Sucrose taken during mixed meal has no additional hyperglycemic action over isocaloric amounts of starch in well-controlled diabetics*, Lancet, 1984, 122-124.

SPRING B., *Psychological effects of carbohydrates*, J. Clin. Psychiatry, 1989, 50-5, suppl., 27-33.

STACH J.K.. *Contribution à l'étude d'une diététique rationnelle du diabétique: rythme circadien de la tolérance au glucose, intérêt pain complet, intérêt du sorbitol*, Thèse pour le doctorat en Médecine, Caen 1974.

TORSDOTTIR I., *Gastric emptying and glycemic response following ingestion of mashed bean or potato flakes in composite meals*, Am. J. Clin. Nutr. Diet, 1990 (sous presse en 1990, cité par Bornet in Cah. Nutr. Diet., 1990, XXV, 4, 254-264).

THORBURN A.W., *The glycemic index of food*, Med. J. Austr., 26 May 1988, 144, 580-582.

VAGUE P., *Influence comparée des différents glucides alimentaires sur la sécrétion hormonale. Les sucres dans l'alimentation*, Collection Scientifique de la Fondation Française pour la Nutrition.

LIPIDS

BOURRE J.M-DURAND G., *The importance of dietary linoleic acid in composition of nervous membranes. Diet and life style, new technology*, De M.F. Mayol, 1988, John Libbey Eurotext Ltd., 477-481.

BOURRE J.M., *Les bonnes graisses*, Ed. Odile Jacob, 1991.

DREON D.M., *The effects of polyunsaturated fat versus mono unsaturated fat on plasma lipoproteins*, JAMA, 1990, 263,

2462-2466.

DYERBER G.J., *Linolenic acid and eicosapentaenoic acid*, Lancet 26 janvier 1980, p. 199.

GUERGUEN L., *Interactions lipides-calcium alimentaires et biodisponibilité du calcium du fromage*, Cah. Nutr. Diet., 1992, XXVII, 5, 311-314.

JACOTOT B., *Olive oil and the lipoprotein metabolism*. Rev. Fr. des Corps Gras, 1988, 2, 5 1-55.

JACOTOT B., *L'huile d'olive, de la santé à la gastronomie*, Ed. Artulen, 1993.

KUSHI, *Diet and 20 years mortality from coronary heart disease*. The Ireland-Boston Diet-Heart study. New England J. of Medicine, 1985, 312, 811-818.

LOUHERANTA A.M., *Linoleic acid intake and susceptibility of VLDL and LDL to oxidation in men*, Am. J. Clin. Nutr., 1996, 63, 698-703.

LOUIS-SYLVESTRE J., *À propos de la consommation actuelle de lipides*, Diétécom, 1996.

MAILLARD C., *Graisses grises*, Gazette Méd. de Fr., 1989, 96, n° 22.

MENSIK R.P., *Effect of dietary fatty acids on high-density and low-density lipoprotein cholesterol levels in healthy*.

ODENT M., *Les acides gras essentiels*, Ed. Jacques Ligier, 1990.

RUASSE J.P., *Des lipides, pourquoi, comment ?* Coll. L'indispensable en nutrition.

SAN JUAN P.M.F., *Study of isomeric trans-fatty acids content in the commercial Spanish foods*, Int. J. of Food Sc. & Nutr., 1996, 47, 399-403.

TROISI R., *Trans-fatty acid intake in relation to serum lipid concentrations in adult men*, Am. J. Clin. Nutr., 1992, 56, 1019-1024.

VLES R.O., *Connaissances récentes sur les effets physiologiques des margarines riches en acide linoléique*, Rev. Fr. des Corps Gras, 1980, 3, 115-120.

WILLETT W.C., *Intake of trans-fatty acids and risk of coronary heart disease among women*, Lancet, 1993, 341, 581-585.

FIBRE

"Council Scientific Affairs" *Fibres alimentaires et santé* JAMA, 1984, 14, 190, 1037-1046.

ANDERSON J.W., *Dietary fiber: diabetes and obesity*, Am. J. Gastroenterology, 1986, 81, 898-906.

BERNIER J.J., *Fibres alimentaires, motricité et absorption intestinale. Effets sur l'hyperglycémie post-prandiale,* Journée de Diabétologie Hôtel-Dieu, 1979, 269-273.

HABER G.B., *Depletion and disruption of dietary fibre. Effects on satiety plasma glucose and serum insulin*, Lancet, 1977, 2, 679-682.

HEATON K.W., *Food fiber as an obstacle to energy intake Lancet*, 1973, 2, 1418-1421.

HEATON K.W., *Dietary fiber in perspective*, Human Clin. Nutr., 1983, 37c, 151-170.

HOLT S., *Effect of gel fibre on gastric emptying and absorption of glucose and paracetamol*, Lancet, 1979, March 24, 636-639.

JENKINS D.J.A., *Decrease in post-prandial insulin and glu-*

cose concentration by guar and pectin, Ann. Int. Med., 1977, 86, 20-33.

JENKINS D.J.A., *Dietary fiber, fibre analogues and glucose tolerance: importance of viscosity*, Br. Med. J., 1978, 1, 1392-1394.

LAURENT B., *Études récentes concernant les fibres alimentaires*, Med. et Nutr., 1983, XIX, 2, 95-122.

MONNIER L., *Effets des fibres sur le métabolisme glucidique*, Cah. Nutr. Diet, 1983, XVIII, 89-93.

NAUSS K.M., *Dietary fat and fiber: relationship to caloric intake body growth and colon carcinogenesis*, Am. J Clin. Nutr., 1987, 45, 243-25 1.

SAUTIER C., *Valeur alimentaire des algues spirulines chez l'homme*, Ann. Nutr. Alim., 1975, 29, 517.

SAUTIER C., *Les algues en alimentation humaine*, Cah. Nutr. Diet, 1987, 6, 469-472.

GENERAL POINTS ON CHOLESTEROL

BASDEVANT A., TRAYNARD P.Y., *Hypercholestérolémie, Symptômes*, 1988, n° 12.

BRUCKERT E., *Les dyslipidémies Impact Médecin* ; Dossier du Praticien n° 20, 1989.

LUC G., DOUSTE-BLAZY P., FRUCHART J.C., *Le cholestérol, d'ou vient-il ? Comment circule-t-il ? Où va-t-il ?*, Rev. Prat 1989, 39, 12, 1011-1017.

POLONOWSKI J., *Régulation de l'absorption intestinale du cholestérol*, Cahiers Nutr. Diet, 1989, 1, 19-25.

LIPIDS & CHOLESTEROL

BETTERIDGE D.J., *High-density lipoprotein and coronary heart disease*, Brit. Med. J., 15 April 1989, 974-975.

DURAND G. et al., *Effets comparés d'huiles végétales et d'huiles de poisson sur le cholestérol du rat*, Med. et Nutr., 1985, XXI, n° 6, 39 1-406.

Consensus: Conference on lowering blood cholesterol to prevent heart disease, JAMA, 1985, 253, 2080-2090.

DYERBERG J. et al., *Eicosapentaenoic acid and prevention of thrombosis and atherosclerosis*. Lancet, 1978, 2, 117-119.

ERNST E., LE MIGNON D., *Les acides gras omega 3 et l'artériosclérose CR de Ther*, 1987, V, n° 56, 22-25.

FIELD C., *The influence of eggs upon plasma cholesterol levels*, Nutr. Rev., 1983, 41, n° 9, 242-244.

FOSSATI P., FERMON C., *Huiles de poisson, intérêt nutritionnel et prévention de l'athéromatose*, Nouv. Presse. Med., 1988, VIII, 1-7.

de GENNES J.L., TURPING. TRFFERT J., *Correction thérapeutique des hyperlipidémies idiopathiques héréditaires. Bilan d'une consultation Consultation de diététique standardisée*, Nouv. Presse Med., 1973, 2, 2457-2464.

GRUNDY M.A., *Comparison of monosaturated fatty acids and carbohydrates for lowering plasma cholesterol*, N. Engl. J. Med., 1986, 314, 745-749.

HAY C.R.M., *Effect of fish oil on platelet kinetics in patients with ischaemic heart disease*, Lancet, 5 June 1982, 1269-1272.

KRUMHOUT D., BOSSCHIETER E.B., LEZENNECOU-LANDER C., *The inverse relation between fish consumption and 20-year mortality from coronary heart disease*, New. Engl. J. Med., 1985, 312, 1205-1209.

LEAF A., WEBER P.C., *Cardiovascular effects of n-3 fatty acids*, New Engl. J. Med., 1988, 318, 549-557.

LEMARCHAL P., *Les acides gras polyinsaturés en Oméga 3*. Cah. Nutr. Diet., 1985, XX, 2, 97-102.

MARINIER E., *Place des acides gras polyinsaturés de la famille n-3 dans le traitement des dysloprotéinémies*, Med. Dig. Nutr., 1986, 53, 14-16.

MARWICK C., *What to do about dietary saturated fats?*, JAMA, 1989, 262, 453.

PHILLIPSON et al., *Reduction of plasma lipids, lipoproteins and apoproteins by dietary fish oils in patients with hypertriglyceridemia*, New Engl. J. Med., 1985, 312, 1210-1216.

PICLET G., *Le poisson, aliment, composition, intérêt nutritionnel*, Cah. Nutr. Diet, 1987, XXII, 3 17-336.

THORNGREN M., *Effects of 11-week increase in dietary eicosapentaenoic acid on bleeding time, lipids and platelet aggregation*, Lancet, 28 Nov. 1981, 1190-11.

TURPIN G., *Régimes et médicaments abaissant la cholestérolémie*, Rev. du Prat., 1989, 39, 12, 1024-1029.

VLES R.O., *Les acides gras essentiels en physiologie cardiovasculaire*, Ann. Nutr. Alim., 1980, 34, 255-264.

WOODCOCK B.E., *Beneficial effect of fish oil on blood viscosity in peripheral vascular disease*, Br. Med. J., Vol. 288, 25 février 1984, p. 592-594.

DIETARY FIBRE & HYPERCHOLESTEROLEMIA

ANDERSON J.W., *Dietary fiber lipids and atherosclerosis*, Am. J. Cardiol., 1987, 60, 17-22.

GIRAULT A., *Effets bénéfiques de la consommation de pommes sur le métabolisme lipidique chez l'homme*, Entretiens de Bichat, 28 septembre 1988.

LEMONNIER D., DOUCET C., FLAMENT C., *Effet du son et de la pectine sur les lipides sériques du rat*, Cah. Nutr. Diet., 1983, XVII, 2, 97.

RAUTUREAU J., COSTE T., KARSENTI P., *Effets des fibres alimentaires sur le métabolisme du cholestérol*, Cah. Nutr. Diet, 1983, XVIII, 2, 84-88.

SABLE-AMPLIS R., SICART R., BARON A., *Influence des fibres de pomme sur le taux d'esters de cholestérol du foie, de l'intestin et de l'aorte*, Cah. Nutr. Diet, 1983, XVII, 2, 97.

TAGLIAFFERRO V. et al., *Moderate guar-gum addition to usual diet improves peripheral sensibility to insulin and lipaemic profile in NIDDM*, Diabète et Métabolisme, 1985, 11, 380-385.

TOGNARELLI M., Guar-pasta: *a new diet for obese subjects*, Acta Diabet. Lat., 1986, 23, 77.

TROWELL H., *Dietary fiber and coronary heart disease*, Europ. J. Clin. Biol. Res., 1972, 17, 345.

VAHOUNY G.U., *Dietary fiber lipid metabolism and atherosclerosis*, Fed. Proc., 1982, 41, 2801-2806.

ZAVOLAL J.H., *Effets hypolipémiques d'aliments contenant du caroube*, Am. J. Clin. Nutr., 1983, 38, 285-294.

VITAMINS, TRACE ELEMENTS & HYPERCHOLESTEROLEMIA

1. Vitamin E

CAREW T.E., *Antiatherogenic effect of probucol unrelated to its hypocholesterolemic effect P.N.A.S.*, USA, June 1984, Vol. 84, 7725-7729.

FRUCHART J.C., *Influence de la qualité des LDL sur leur métabolisme et leur arthérogénicité* (unpublished).

JURGENS G., *Modification of human serum LDL by oxydation, Chemistry and Physics of Lipids*, 1987, 45, 315-336.

STREINBRECHER V.P., *Modifications of LDL by endothelial cells involves lipid peroxydation P.N.A.S.*, USA, June 1984, Vol. 81, 3883-3887.

2. Selenium

LUOMA P.V., *Serum selenium, glutathione peroxidase, lipids, and human liver microsomal enzyme activity, Biological Trace Element Research*, 1985, 2, 8, 113-121.

MITCINSON M.J., *Possible role of deficiency of selenium and vitamin E in atherosclerosis*, J. Clin. Pathol., 1984, 37, 7-837.

SALONEN J.T., *Serum fatty acids, apolipoproteins, selenium and vitamin antioxydants and risk of death from coronary artery disease*, Am. J. Cardiol., 1985, 56, 4, 226-23 1.

3. Chromium

ABRAHAM A.S., *The effect of chromium established atherosclerotic plaques in rabbits*, Am. J. Clin. Nutr., 1980, 33, 2294-2298.

GORDON T., *High-density lipoprotein as a protective factor against coronary heart disease*, The Framingham Study, Am. J. Med., 1977, 62, 707.

OFFENBACHER E.G., *Effect of chromium-rich yeast on glucose tolerance of blood lipids in elderly subjects*, Diabetes, 1980, 29, 919-925.

COFFEE & HYPERCHOLESTEROLEMIA

ARNESEN E., *Coffee and serum cholesterol*, Br. Med. J., 1984, 288, 1960.

HERBERT P.N., *Caffeine does not affect lipoprotein metabolism*, Clin. Res., 1987, 35, 578A.

HILL C., *Coffee consumption and cholesterol concentration*, Letter to editor, Br. Med. J., 1985, 290, 1590.

THELLE D.S., *Coffee and cholesterol in epidemiological and experimental studies*, Atherosclerosis, 1987, 67, 97-103.

THELLE D.S., *The Tromso Heart Study. Does coffee raise serum cholesterol?*, N. Engl. J. Med., 1983, 308, 1454-1457.

GENERAL POINTS ON OBESITY

ADRIAN F., *Divergent trends in obesity and fat intake pattern:the American paradox*, Am. J. Med., 1997, 102, 259-264.

ASTIER-DUMAS M., *Densité calorique, densité nutritionnelle, repères pour le choix des aliments*, Med. Nutr. 1984, XX, 4, 229-234.

BOUCHARD C., *Génétique et métabolisme énergétique chez l'homme*. In Forum Lavoisier, Paris, 1989.

BELLISLE F., *Obesity and food intake in children: evidence for a role of metabolic and/or behavioral daily rhythms*, Appetite, 1988, 11, 111-118.

BROWNELL K.D., *The effects of repeated cycles of weight loss and regain in rats*, Phys. Behaviour, 1986, 38, 459-464.

FRICKER J., APFELBAUM M., *Le métabolisme de l'obésité* - La Recherche, 1989, 20, 207, 200-208.

HERAUD G., *Densité nutritionnelle des aliments*, Gaz. Med. Fr., 1988, 95, 13, 39-42.

HILLS A.P., WAHLQUIST M.L., *Exercise and obesity*, Ed. Smith-Gordon, 1994.

LEIBEL R.J., *Diminished energy requirements in reduced obese persons*, Metabolism, 1984, 33, 164-170.

LOUIS-SYLVESTRE J., *Consommation d'un plat allégé et répercussion sur la prise alimentaire totale*. Le Généraliste, 1979, 1083.

RIETVELD W.J., *L'horloge biologique*. Revue de nutrition, Diétécom, 1991, 80.

ROLLAND-CACHERA M.F., BELLISLE F., *No correlation between adiposity and food intake: why are working class children fatter?* Am. J. Clin. Nutr., 1986, 44, 779-787.

ROLAND-CACHERA M.F., DEHEEGER M., *Adiposity and food intake in young children: the environmental challenge to individual susceptibility*, Br. Med. J., 1988, 296, 1037-1038.

ROLLAND-CACHERA M.F., *La France est-elle privilégiée par rapport aux autres pays développés ?* 1ère journées alimentation, kilos, santé, 1997.

RUASSE J.P, *Des calories, pourquoi ? Combien ?*, Coll. L'indispensable en nutrition, 1987.

RUASSE J.P., *L'approche homéopathique du traitement des obésités*, Paris, 1988.

SPITZER L., RODIN J., *Human eating behavior: a critical review of studies in normal weight and overweight individuals*, Appetite, 1981, 2, 293.

LOUIS-SYLVESTRE J., *Poids accordéon : de plus en plus difficile à perdre*, Le Gén., 1989, 1087, 18-20.

DIETARY HABITS

HERCBERG S., *Apports nutritionnels d'un échantillon représentatif de la population du Val de Marne*, Rev. Epidem. et Santé Publ., 1991, 39.

MARCOCCHIN N., *Comportement alimentaire en Lorraine, Précis de nutrition et diététique*, fasc. 10, Pub. Ardix Médical.

RIGAUD D. et coll., *Enquête de consommation alimentaire I - Energie et macronutriments*, Cah. Nutr. Diet., 1997, 32, 6, 379-389.

INSULIN

BASDEVANT A., *Influence de la distribution de la masse grasse sur le risque vasculaire*, La Presse Médicale, 1987, 16, 4.

CLARK M.G., *Obesity with insulin resistance*. Experimental insights, Lancet, 1983, 2, 1236-1240.

DANGUIR J., *Infusion of insulin causes relative increase of slow wave sleep in rats*. Brain Research, 1984, 306, 97-103.

FROMAN L.A., *Effect of vagotomy and vagal stimulation on insulin secretion*, Diabetes, 1967, 16, 443-448.

GROSS P., *De l'obésité au diabète,* L'actualité diabétologique, n° 13, P. 1-9.

GUY-GRAND B., *Variation des acides gras libres plasmatiques au cours des hyperglycémies provoquées par voie orale,* Journées de Diabétologie de l'Hôtel-Dieu, 1968, p. 319.

GUY-GRAND B., *Rôle éventuel du tissu adipeux dans l'insulinorésistance,* Journées de Diabétologie de l'Hôtel-Dieu, 1972, 81-92.

JEANRENAUD B., *Dysfonctionnement du système nerveux. Obésité et résistance à l'insuline,* M/S Médecine-Science, 1987, 3, 403-410.

JEANRENAUD B., *Insulin and obesity,* Diabetologia, 1979, 17, 135-138.

KOLTERMAN O.G., *Mechanisms of insulin resistance in human obesity. Evidence for receptor and post-receptor effects,* J. Clin. Invest., 1980, 65, 1272-1284.

LAMBERT A.F., *Enhancement by caffeine of glucagon-inducet and tolbutamide induced insulin release from isolated foetal pancreatic tissue,* Lancet, 1967, 1, 1, 19, 819-820.

LAMBERT A.E., *Organocultures de pancréas foetal de rat: étude morphologique et libération d'insuline in vitro,* Journées de Diabétologie de l'Hôtel-Dieu, 1969, 115-129.

LARSON B., *Abdominal adipose tissue distribution, obesity and risk of cardio-vascular disease and death,* Br. Med. J., 1984, 288, 1401-1404.

LE MARCHAND-BRUSTEL Y., *Résistance à l'insuline dans l'obésité*, M/S Médecine-Sciences 1987, 3, 394-402.

LINQUETTE C., *Précis d'endocrinologie*, Ed. Masson, 1973, 658- 666.

LOUIS-SYLVESTRE J., *La phase céphalique de sécrétion d'insuline*, Diabète et métabolisme, 1987, 13, 63-73.

MARKS V., *Action de différents stimuli sur l'insulinosécrétion humaine : influence du tractus gastro-intestinal*, Journées de Diabétologie de l'Hôtel-Dieu, 1969, 179-190.

MARLISSE E.B., *Système nerveux central et glycorégulation*, Journées de Diabétologie de l'Hôtel-Dieu, 1975, 7-21.

MEYLAN M., *Metabolic factors in insulin resistance in human obesity*, Metabolism, 1987, 36, 256-261.

WOODS S.C., *Interaction entre l'insulinosécrétion et le système nerveux central*, Journées de Diabétologie de l'Hôtel-Dieu, 1983.

DIABETICS

American Diabetes Association, *Clinical practice recommendations*, Diabetes Care, 1995, 18, suppl. 1, 16-19.

ANDERSEN E., *Effect of rice-rich versus a potato-rich diet on glucose, lipoprotein and cholesterol metabolism in noninsulindependent diabetics*, Am. J. Clin., Nutr., 1984, 39, 598-606.

BORNET F., *Insulinemic and glycemic indexes of six starchrich foods taken alone and in a mixed meal by type 2 diabetic*, Am. J. Clin. Nutr., 1987, 45, 588-595.

BORNET F., *Technologie des amidons, digestibilité et effets métaboliques*, Cah. Nutr. Diet., 1992, 27, 170-178.

BRAND-MILLER J.C., *Importance of glycemic index in diabe-*

tes, Am. J Clin. Nutr., 1994, 59 suppl., 747 S-752 S.

BRAND-MILLER J.C., The G.I. factor: *the glycemic index solution. The scientific answer to weight reduction and blood sugar control*, A Holder & Stroughton Book, Australia, 1997.

FONTVIEILLE A.M., *A moderate switch from high to low glycemic-index foods for 3 weeks improves the metabolic control of type I diabetic subjects*, Diab. Nutr. Metab., 1988, 1, 139- 143.

JENKINS D.J.A., *Glycemic index of foods : a physiological basis for carbohydrate exchange*, Am. J. Clin. Nutr., 1981, 34, 362- 366.

JENKINS D.J.A., *Metabolic effects of low-glycemic index diet*, Am. J. Clin. Nutr., 1987, 46, 968-975.

JENKINS D.J.A., *Low glycemic index; lente carbohydrates and physiological effects of altered food frequency*, Am. J. Clin. Nutr., 1994, 56 suppl., 706 S-709 S.

LORMEAU B., VALENSI P., *L'alimentation du diabétique*, Cah. Nutr. Diet., 1997, 32, 6, 394-400.

MONNIER L., SLAMA G., *Recommandations ALFEDIAM*, Diabetes Metabolism, 1995, 21, 201-217.

Nutritional recommendations and principles for individuals with diabetes mellitus, Diabetes care, 1990, 13, suppl. I, 18-25.

O'DEA K., *Physical factors influency post-prandial glucose and insulin responses to starch*, Am. J. Clin. Nutr., 1980, 33, 760- 765.

SIMPSON H.C.R., *A high carbohydrate leguminous fibre diet improves all aspects of diabetic control*, Lancet, 1981, 1, 1-5.

SLAMA G., *Diabete : conseils nutritionnels,* Impact Médecin Hebdo, 13 juin 1997, n° 370, 5 1-53.

PHYSICAL ACTIVITY & EXERCISE

BLAIR D., *Habitual daily energy expenditure and activity levels of lean and adult-onset and child-onset obese women*, Am. J. Clin. Nutr., 1987, 45, 540-550.

BLAIR S.N., *Evidence for success of exercise in weight loss and control*, Annals of Int. Med., 1993, 119, 7, 2; 702-706.

DESPRES J.P., *Obésité abdominale et lipoprotéines : effets de l'exercice*, Science et Sports, 1991, 6, 265-273.

DESPRES J.P., *L'exercice physique dans le traitement de l'obésité*, Cah. Nutr. Diet., 1994, XXIX, 5, 299-304.

GUEZENNEC C.Y., *Place de l'entraînement dans le traitement desmaladiesmétaboliques*,Cah.Nutr.Diet.,1994,XXIX,1,28-37.

KEMPEN K.P.G., *Energy balance during an 8-week energy restricted diet with and without exercise in obese women*, Am. J. Clin. Nutr., 1995, 62, 722-729.

LOUIS SYLVESTRE J., *Insuline et exercice physique*. Diabète et Métabolisme, 1987, 13, 152-156.

MONDENARD de J.P., *Poids et sport. Précis de Nutrition et Diététique*, Fasc. 17, Ardix Médical, 1989.

MARCONNET P., *Effort musculaire et substrats énergétiques*, Cah. Nutr. Diet., 1986, XXI, 2, 109-122.

TREMBLAY A., *Exercice et obésité*, Science et Sports, 1991, 6, 257-264.

WOLF L.M., *Contribution de l'exercice physique au traitement de l'obésité*, Cah. Nutr. Diet, 1986, XXI, 2, 137-141.

WOOD P.D., *The effects on plasma lipoproteins of a prudent weight-reducing diet, with or without exercise, in overweight men and women*, N. Engl. J. Med., 1991, 325, 461-466.

HYPOGLYCEMIA

CAHILL G.F., *A non editorial on non hypoglycemia*, N. Engl. J. Med., 1974, 291, 905-906.

CATHELINEAU G., *Effect of calcium infusion on post reactive hypoglycemia*, Horm. Metab. Res., 1981, 13, 646-647.

CHILES R., *Excessive serum insulin response to oral glucose in obesity and mild diabetes*, Diabetes, 1970, 19, 458.

CRAPO P.A., *The effects of oral fructose, sucrose and glucose in subjects with reactive hypoglycemia*, Diabetes Care, 1982, 5, 5 12-5 17.

DORNER M., *Les hypoglycémies fonctionnelles,* Rev. Prat., 1972, 22, 25, 3427-3446.

FAJANS S.S., *Fasting hypoglycemia in adults*, New Engl. J. Med., 1976, 294, 766-772.

FARRYKANT M., *The problem of functional hyperinsulinism or functional hypoglycemia attributed to nervous causes*, Metabolism, 1971, 20, 6, 428-434.

FIELD J.B., *Studies on the mechanisms of ethanol induced hypoglycemia*, J. Clin. Invest., 1963, 42, 497-506.

FREINKEL N., *Alcohol hypoglycemia*, J. Clin. Invest., 1963, 42, 1112-1133.

HARRIS S., *Hyperinsulinism and dysinsulinism*, JAMA, 1924, 83, 729-733.

HAUTECOUVERTURE M., *Les hypoglycémies fonctionnelles*, Rev. Prat., 1985, 35, 31, 1901-1907.

HOFELDT F.D., *Reactive hypoglycemia*, Metabolism, 1975, 24, 1193-1208.

HOFELDT F.D., *Are abnormalities in insulin secretion respon-*

sible for reactive hypoglycemia?, Diabetes, 1974, 23, 589-596.

JENKINS D.J.A., *Decrease in post-prandial insulin and gluco-se concentrations by guar and pectin*, Ann. Intern. Med., 1977, 86, 20-23.

JOHNSON D.D., *Réactive hypoglycemia*, JAMA, 1980, 243, 115 1-1155.

JUNG Y., *Reactive hypoglycemia in women*, Diabetes, 1971, 20, 428-434.

LEFEBVRE P., *Statement on post-prandial hypoglycemia*, Diabetes Care, 1988, 11, 439-440.

LEFEBVRE P., *Le syndrome d'hypoglycémie réactionnelle, mythe ou réalité ?*, Journées Annuelles de l'Hôtel-Dieu, 1983, 111- 118.

LEICHTER S.B., *Alimentary hypoglycemia: a new appraisal*, Amer. J. Nutr., 1979, 32, 2104-2114.

LEV-RAN A., *The diagnosis of post-prandial hypoglycemia*, Diabetes, 1981, 30, 996-999.

LUBETZKI J., *Physiopathologie des hypoglycémies*, Rev. Prat., 1972, 22, 25, 333 1-3347.

LUYCKY A.S., *Plasma insulin in reactive hypoglycemia*, Diabetes, 1971, 20, 435-442.

MONNIER L.H., *Restored synergistic entero-hormonal res-ponse after addition dietary fibre to patients with impaired glu-cose tolerance and reactive hypoglycemia*, Diab. Metab., 1982, 8, 217-222.

O'KEEFE S.J.D., *Lunch time gin and tonic: a cause of reactive hypoglycemia*, Lancet, 1977, 1, June 18, 1286-1288.

PERRAULT M., *Le régime de fond des hypoglycémies fonc-tionnelles de l'adulte*, Rev. Prat., 1963, 13, 4025-4030.

SENG G., *Mécanismes et conséquences des hypoglycémies*, Rev. Prat., 1985, 35, 31, 1859-1866.

SERVICE J.F., *Hypoglycemia and the post-prandial syndrome*, New Engl., J. Med., 1989, 321, 1472.

SUSSMAN K.E., *Plasma insulin levels during reactive hypoglycemia*, Diabetes, 1966, 15, 1-14.

TAMBURRANO G., *Increased insulin sensitivity in patients with idiopathic reactive hypoglycemia*, J. Clin. Endocr. Metab., 1989, 69, 885.

TAYLOR S.I., *Hypoglycemia associated with antibodies to the insulin receptor*, New. Engl. J. Med., 1982, 307, 1422-1426.

YALOW R.S., *Dynamics of insulin secretion in hypoglycemia*, Diabetes, 1965, 14, 341-350.

NOTES

In our collection Alpen éditions:

-The Omega-3 Answer

-Living with a Hyperactive Child

-All About the Prostate

-The French Paradox

-The XXL Syndrome

with Michel Montignac:

-Eat Yourself Slim

-The Montignac Diet Cookbook

-The French GI Diet

-Glycemic Index Diet

www.alpen.mc